BRAINWASHED
by Your
GUT

Dr Manjari Chandra is a seasoned nutritionist and functional medicine expert with over 25 years of experience. She has served as a senior consultant at Max Healthcare and Manipal Hospitals, in using nutrition to manage and reverse chronic conditions such as diabetes, heart disease, hormonal imbalances, and cancer.

Dr Chandra is the author of *Eat Up Clean Up* and *Heal with Foods*, a regular media contributor on *NDTV* and *India Today*, and writes for *The Times of India* and *Men's Health*. She also conducts workshops across India to promote preventive health and wellness.

BRAINWASHED
by Your
GUT

THE SECRET LINK BETWEEN FOOD AND MOOD

MANJARI CHANDRA

Published by
Rupa Publications India Pvt. Ltd 2025
161-B/4, Gulmohar House,
Yusuf Sarai Community Centre,
New Delhi 110049

Sales centres:
Bengaluru Chennai
Hyderabad Kolkata Mumbai

Copyright © Manjari Chandra 2025

The views and opinions expressed in this book are the author's own and the facts are as reported by her; these have been verified to the extent possible, and the publishers are not in any way liable for the same.

All rights reserved.

No part of this publication may be reproduced, transmitted, or stored in a retrieval system, in any form or by any means, electronic, mechanical, photocopying, recording or otherwise, without the prior permission of the publisher.

P-ISBN: 978-93-7003-469-3
E-ISBN: 978-93-7003-497-6

Third impression 2026

10 9 8 7 6 5 4 3

The moral right of the author has been asserted.

Printed in India

This book is sold subject to the condition that it shall not, by way of trade or otherwise, be lent, resold, hired out, or otherwise circulated, without the publisher's prior consent, in any form of binding or cover other than that in which it is published.

To my patients, whose unwavering faith and relentless pursuit of health have been my greatest source of inspiration, I dedicate this journey to you—your resilience has shaped every word within these pages.

To my mentors, whose wisdom and guidance have illuminated my path, I owe the deepest gratitude for nurturing my passion into purpose.

And to my teachers, whose knowledge and kindness have been the foundation of my growth, I honour you with every lesson shared in this book.

Contents

Foreword ix

Note from the Author xi

Part 1: Connecting the Dots: Food, Gut, Brain and Mental Health 1

1. The Gut-Brain Axis and Mental Health 10
2. Understanding Leaky Gut: Why Food for Our Microbiome Matters 31
3. Stress and the Gut: How Our Environment Affects Our Microbiome 49
4. What Happens When We 'Kill' Our Gut Feeling? 61

Part 2: Healing from Within: Building a Healthier Relationship with Food 79

5. Heal Your Gut, Heal Your Mind: A Plate Full of Prebiotics and Probiotics 86
6. Nourishing the Brain: Foods That Support Neurotransmitters 116
7. The Elimination Protocol: A Path to Optimal Health 148
8. Mindful Eating: Transforming How You Eat 184
9. Intuitive Eating: Awakening the Body's Wisdom 196

A Few Last Words 206
Acknowledgements 209
Index 211

Foreword

As someone who has spent decades working with individuals grappling with mental health issues, I am both humbled and deeply heartened by the direction this book takes. In a world where the mind and body are often treated as separate entities, it is rare to find a resource that so eloquently bridges the two, acknowledging the profound interconnectedness between what we eat and how we feel. *Brainwashed by Your Gut* by Dr Manjari Chandra, a prominent nutritionist, brings this intricate connection to light with the clarity, compassion and evidence-based research it deserves. Mental health is much more than a chemical imbalance or a singular diagnosis; it is the cumulative result of many factors—environmental, emotional and, importantly, nutritional. Our food choices and eating habits shape not only our physical health but also the very functioning of our minds. As a psychiatrist, I have witnessed firsthand the toll that nutritional deficiencies and poor eating habits can take on mental well-being. In my practice, I often wished for a deeper exploration of how food can serve as a potent form of medicine. This book is precisely that—a holistic approach that empowers individuals to harness the power of nutrition to support their emotional and mental health. In each chapter, Dr Chandra takes the reader on a transformative journey, combining solid, evidence-based research with practical advice that can be applied to daily life. More than just a resource for those facing mental health challenges, this book is for anyone who seeks to understand the profound impact of food choices on their mental state. Dr Chandra offers a compassionate and insightful guide to making informed decisions that positively influence mental clarity, emotional stability and overall well-being. As a psychiatrist, it is personally satisfying to see this holistic approach presented in such a comprehensive and eloquent form. Too often, we overlook the significance of simple, everyday acts—like choosing what we eat—and their lasting impact on our mental health. This book offers us the opportunity to step back, re-evaluate, and take control of our well-being in a way that is both empowering and deeply restorative. I encourage every reader to approach this book with an open mind and a sense of curiosity. Let it serve as a reminder that healing can—and should—come from the most fundamental aspects of our lives. Through *Brainwashed by Your Gut*, Dr Chandra has given us a gift, a lifeline with the potential to change lives. I believe this book will become an invaluable resource for anyone seeking not just to survive, but to thrive.

Prof. (Dr) Nimesh G. Desai
Senior Consultant, Psychiatrist and Psychotherapist
Former Director, IHBAS, Delhi
Former Member Secretary/CEO, SMHA, Delhi
President, Manovikas Charitable Society

Note from the Author

As I sit down to write this note, I am filled with a profound sense of excitement, hope and purpose. *Brainwashed by Your Gut* is the culmination of years of professional exploration and personal experiences—an effort to uncover the intricate relationship between our food choices, eating habits and mental health. Writing this book has been deeply personal, shaped not only by my career as a nutritionist but also by a poignant family experience that reshaped my understanding of mental well-being.

The seeds of this book were sown early in my career when I noticed a recurring pattern among my clients. Many, despite following conventional dietary advice, continued to struggle with anxiety, depression and challenges to their overall mental well-being. It became clear that the equation was far more complex than simply counting calories, macros or vitamins. This observation led me to ask: *Could there be a deeper, intrinsic link between the nutrients we consume and our psychological health?* My journey as a nutritionist inspired me to uncover the truth about how what we eat profoundly influences how we feel.

Over the years, I have observed a troubling rise in mental health issues that are not necessarily tied to catastrophic personal or financial losses, but rather to everyday lifestyle choices. This subtle yet profound form of distress—often overlooked—quietly diminishes the quality of life for many. It is this form of mental health struggle that I am determined to address through the pages of this book.

This book bridges the gap between scientific research and practical, everyday living. It is for anyone who has ever wondered how their diet affects their mood, for those seeking a more holistic approach to mental well-being, and for individuals who believe in the healing power of food. My hope is that through this book, you will gain a deeper understanding of how to harness nutrition to support your emotional and mental health. Each chapter blends evidence-based research with practical strategies, offering tools to make informed food choices that positively impact mental well-being. You will learn about the gut-brain axis, the role of the gut microbiome in neurotransmitter production, and the connection between food and mental states. I also explore how a compromised gut barrier, commonly known as a 'leaky gut', is linked to various mental health disorders. A significant focus is placed on key neurotransmitters—dopamine, oxytocin, serotonin and endorphins—and their role in emotional stability. Additionally, I highlight specific nutrients that support brain health and discuss how mindful and intuitive eating can transform our relationship with food.

Despite growing scientific evidence, the role of diet in mental health remains underexplored in mainstream discussions. Through this book, I hope to initiate a shift in how we approach mental health treatment—integrating nutrition as a fundamental pillar of healing.

I write this book not only as a nutritionist but also as a mother, wife and daughter who has witnessed firsthand the transformative power of food in enhancing well-being. My father's journey from despair to hope through dietary changes has been my greatest motivation. His experience reinforced my belief that the right nutrition can be life-changing. With the **rise in mental health disorders**, statistics show that **one in five Indians** experiences symptoms of mental illness. Globally, the number of people suffering from **depressive symptoms** surged from **193 million before the pandemic to 246 million in the post-Covid period**.[1] One emerging area of study is the link between **leaky gut and mental health**—a concept I explore in depth throughout this book.

I have divided this book into two major parts, each comprising four chapters. The first part addresses the prevailing issue of declining mental health, beginning with an introduction to the gut-brain axis and its significance in ensuring overall well-being. It highlights the bidirectional communication between the gut and the brain, emphasizing the gut's role in influencing mood, cognition and behaviour. The discussion then shifts to how certain dietary patterns contribute to mental health ailments. Many common diets exacerbate conditions such as anxiety, depression and mood swings, often due to the detrimental effects of processed foods, excessive sugars and unhealthy fats on brain function. By identifying these dietary culprits, we can begin to understand the urgency of finding solutions to these problems.

Another crucial aspect I explore is the impact of stress on mental health. Psychological stress triggers the release of cortisol, the body's primary stress hormone, which plays a key role in our response to external pressures. However, prolonged stress and elevated cortisol levels lead to dysregulation, contributing to anxiety disorders, depression and cognitive impairments. Chronic stress also affects gut permeability, leading to systemic inflammation that disrupts brain function. This brings us to

---

[1] Jain, R., 'World Mental Health Day: 60-70 mn people in India suffer from common mental disorders; stigmatization & financial barriers prevent timely treatment', *The Economic Times*, 10 October 2023, https://tinyurl.com/r8bymr85. Accessed on 13 March 2025.

the concept of 'leaky gut'—a condition where the integrity of the gut lining is compromised, allowing harmful substances to enter the bloodstream and contribute to neuroinflammation. Understanding this connection is critical to addressing mental health from a holistic perspective.

The second part of this book offers practical solutions to enhance mental well-being through dietary interventions and mindful eating. I explore the role of prebiotics, probiotics and neurotransmitter-boosting nutrients in restoring gut health and mental clarity. These foods do more than just nourish the body—they actively support the gut-brain axis and ensure the optimal functioning of brain chemistry. Through a comprehensive examination of recent scientific research, I illustrate how nutrients such as omega-3 fatty acids, B vitamins and antioxidants play essential roles in maintaining mental health—influencing everything from neurotransmitter production to the inflammation levels in the brain. For many of my clients, these insights have been transformative—simple yet powerful dietary changes led to significant improvements in their mental states.

Beyond specific foods, I introduce the concepts of mindful eating and intuitive eating. Mindful eating encourages us to fully engage with the sensory experience of food, cultivating a healthier relationship with eating and reducing emotional triggers. Intuitive eating, on the other hand, promotes an internal, body-led approach to nourishment by tuning into hunger and satiety signals. Both of these practices offer a sustainable, balanced way to reconnect with food in a way that enhances our mental well-being.

To help integrate these principles into daily life, I provide practical guidelines on mindful and intuitive eating—how to create a conducive eating environment, engage the senses, and develop a heightened awareness of food choices. By adopting these practices, we can transform our eating habits and, in turn, our mental health.

This book is the culmination of my quest to share these insights with a broader audience. It is designed for anyone who feels trapped in the throes of lifestyle-induced depression, and seeks a natural, sustainable way to regain their mental balance. It provides a comprehensive guide to understanding how different foods affect mood and mental health, supported by the latest scientific research and practical advice on implementing these changes in everyday life.

By blending nutritional science with mindfulness, this book presents a sustainable, natural approach to supporting mental health, reducing stress and preventing disorders. The strategies outlined here are not about drastic overhauls, but about making informed, mindful choices that nourish both body and mind. From understanding the importance of gut health to learning which nutrients are essential for mental clarity and emotional stability, this book equips you with the knowledge and tools to take control of your mental well-being through your diet.

Thank you for allowing me to share this journey with you. May this book serve as a guide and companion as you explore the powerful connection between what you eat and how your mind functions.

PART 1

Connecting the Dots: Food, Gut, Brain and Mental Health

There were days when 'Sarah'[1] would break into tears without warning. She often told me how she lashed out at others when, in reality, she wanted to scream at herself. *At herself?* I found myself wondering. After all, she had a promising start to her career—appointed as a senior-level manager in her very first job. Everything seemed set for a dream run. Yet there she was—withdrawn, burdened, and unable to understand why.

The roots of her depression were planted early in her professional journey. Sarah, a young MBA graduate from one of India's top 10 colleges, secured a senior position straight out of university. It was a remarkable achievement, but instead of feeling triumphant, she felt scrutinized. She believed that some colleagues resented her rapid rise though she couldn't be certain whether it was real or perceived.

She once confided in me that she felt invisible, as if the only way to be acknowledged was to be *exceptionally* charming. She dressed impeccably, forced herself to be an extrovert, and maintained a friendly, approachable demeanour with everyone—colleagues, juniors and seniors alike. On social media, she curated an image of confidence and success, posting carefully selected photos accompanied by motivational captions. But after months of this, she began to feel as though she were begging for validation. The realization that she needed external approval to feel worthy left her feeling hollow.

It wasn't that Sarah lacked appreciation. Her bosses praised her and she received positive engagement on social media. Yet self-doubt had taken root—convincing her that she was *not enough* on her own, that her talent alone was insufficient, and that without this carefully maintained image, she would go unnoticed

---

[1] The patient's name has been changed for privacy.

or unappreciated. That thought made her profoundly unhappy.

Sarah was struggling with self-esteem issues.

She attended office parties, dined with colleagues and participated in workplace social events. Yet, the moment she left the office, an overwhelming loneliness set in. The more she immersed herself in social activities, the more acutely she felt the emptiness afterwards—an unsettling silence that seemed to seep into her. But was she truly alone? When I probed further, I found that she had a close group of friends—people she could have confided in and been her true self with. Yet she chose to distance herself from them, investing all her energy in seeking approval from her colleagues instead.

When she didn't receive the validation she craved, the carefully constructed façade collapsed. It wasn't that she was dishonest—rather, she was trying to become someone she wasn't, and for no real reason. The frustration she once masked with cheerfulness turned into unchecked resentment. She snapped at colleagues, particularly those in senior and junior positions. She became irritable over the smallest instructions from her bosses. As things spiralled downwards, she would return home feeling defeated, crying uncontrollably—convinced that she failed, fearful of losing her job, and unsure of how to *fix* things.

Her disappointment soon turned into withdrawal. She stopped dining with colleagues, skipped office parties, and even began standing at the farthest corner of the room during workplace celebrations, reluctant to engage. She was ashamed of her struggles, unwilling to open up about her emotions, and cut herself off from family and friends. This pattern, unfortunately, is all too common in cases of depression.

Sarah wasn't just struggling with workplace stress—she was lost in a cycle of self-doubt and emotional exhaustion. Of course, external circumstances played a role in it, but such challenges are not uncommon in professional environments. The difference lies in how individuals cope. Some develop **internal resilience**, adapting and finding ways to regain control. Others rely on **strong support systems**—friends and family who provide comfort and perspective. But those who lack both are the most vulnerable.

Over time, our understanding of mental health has evolved significantly—shaped by cultural, scientific and societal advancements. In ancient civilizations, mental illness was often attributed to supernatural or divine forces. The Mesopotamians, Egyptians and Greeks believed disorders were manifestations of divine displeasure or demonic possession, leading to treatments such as exorcisms and prayers. In ancient India, however, Ayurveda took a more holistic approach. Ayurvedic texts emphasized that mental well-being was deeply intertwined with diet, lifestyle and emotional balance. These early beliefs laid the foundation for perspectives that persisted across generations, influencing cultural attitudes towards mental health.

Ayurvedic dietary principles stress the importance of consuming fresh, seasonal and locally sourced foods to maintain both physical and mental equilibrium. Certain foods and spices are revered for their ability to pacify or aggravate specific *dosha*s and influence mental states. Warm, home-cooked meals enriched with turmeric, ginger and cinnamon are believed to promote digestion, vitality and emotional stability. In contrast, excessive consumption of processed foods, stimulants and heavy, difficult-to-digest foods is thought to impair gut function, leading to mental fog, lethargy and emotional instability.

Modern research increasingly aligns with these ancient principles, revealing that what we eat directly impacts neurotransmitter function, gut health and overall mental well-being. The foods we consume either nourish or deplete our cognitive and emotional resilience. And as Sarah's story illustrates, the consequences of neglecting this connection can be profound.

> Hi there, 🙋
>
> I am Social Media; I have been making some noise lately on the importance of mental health and well-being. I have lent voices to so many people now that it is difficult to filter out misinformation and frivolous opinions of influencers from facts and experiential insights of experts.
>
> And it is unfortunate! 😊
>
> This is why it is important to read this book thoroughly—to cut the noise. For starters, Part 1 discusses the role of the gut in optimizing mental health, and why the gut-brain connection needs to be seriously addressed when it comes to understanding and treating mental health ailments. By the time you finish reading Part 1, you will have understood how the food we eat manifests mental health issues by affecting the gut-brain connection. And that is when I will see you again in Part 2!

In recent years, mental health has emerged as a significant global concern, with increasing attention being paid to the prevalence and impact of mental health disorders across the world. From depression and anxiety to schizophrenia and bipolar disorder—these conditions affect individuals of all ages and backgrounds. A report from the World Health Organization (WHO) highlighted a massive 25 per cent increase in the prevalence of anxiety and depression during the Covid-19 pandemic, with youngsters and women being worst hit. And it becomes more worrisome when we consider this information as just the tip of the iceberg.

According to WHO, mental health disorders represent one of the leading causes of disability worldwide. The Global Burden of Disease study (2019) estimated that mental and substance use disorders accounted for approximately 16 per cent of the global burden of disease,[2] surpassing both cardiovascular diseases (CVDs) and cancer in terms of disability-adjusted life years (DALYs) lost. In simpler terms, people suffering from mental health disorders are expected to lose more years of their lives compared to those suffering from CVD or cancer. This staggering statistic underscores the profound impact of mental health disorders on individuals, families and societies.

A recent study published in 2022 has shown that mental disorders increased by 48.1 per cent between 1991 and 2019.[3]

Worldwide, the number of people suffering from depressive symptoms has risen from 193 million before the Covid-19 pandemic to 246 million in the post-Covid period. With the continuous rise in cases of mental disorder, analyses have shown that one in every five individuals suffers from some or the other form of mental illness.

In India, the numbers are alarming—close to 60–70 million people are suffering from some form of mental disorder,[4]

---

[2] Arias, D., S. Saxena, and S. Verguet, 'Quantifying the global burden of mental disorders and their economic value', *eClinicalMedicine*, Vol. 54, 101675, 2022, https://tinyurl.com/ymeujba4. Accessed on 13 March 2025.

[3] GBD 2019 Mental Disorders Collaborators, 'Global, regional, and national burden of 12 mental disorders in 204 countries and territories, 1990–2019: a systematic analysis for the Global Burden of Disease Study 2019', *The Lancet Psychiatry*, Vol. 9, No. 2, 2022, pp. 137–150, https://tinyurl.com/4chpzjsw. Accessed on 13 March 2025.

[4] Jain, R., 'World Mental Health Day'.

*with its suicide rate at one of its highest levels
in history since we started recording it.*

It is apparent that today, too many people remain without access to the care and support they need for both pre-existing and newly developed mental health conditions. This is why in its report, WHO has urged mental health advocates to change their attitudes, actions and approaches to mental health and its care. One such approach is to monitor and target gut health. To do that, we must acknowledge the intensity of the connection that the gastrointestinal tract (gut) shares with the brain. The gut is embedded with microorganisms, mainly bacteria of numerous groups—collectively referred to as **gut microbiota**. Gut microbes enable the gut to form links that influence many bodily organs to various degrees, the most important of which is with the brain. This is called the **gut-brain axis,** which we will address in the upcoming chapters.

One emerging area in recent studies is the potential impact of a condition known as **'leaky gut'** on mental health. Under normal circumstances, the intestinal lining acts as a barrier—selectively permitting nutrients to pass through while keeping harmful substances at bay. However, when the intestinal lining becomes more porous than usual, it allows toxins, microbes and undigested food particles to leak into the bloodstream, giving the phenomenon its name.

The gut produces an array of neurotransmitters, including serotonin, dopamine and gamma-aminobutyric acid (GABA), which play crucial roles in regulating mood, behaviour and cognition. Disruptions in gut permeability due to leaky gut can compromise the synthesis and signalling of neurotransmitters, potentially precipitating mood disturbances and cognitive impairments—highlighting the significance of gastrointestinal health in modulating serotonin levels and mood stability.

> *More than 50 per cent of the dopamine and 90 per cent of the serotonin in our bodies is produced in the gut,[5] and these neurotransmitters are transmitted to the brain via the gut-brain axis.*

So, what is causing a leaky gut and poor mental health symptoms? At the forefront is the sugar-rich, industrially processed or substandard quality of the food we eat.

Our gut is home to both good and pathogenic bacteria. Good bacteria (probiotics) thrive on foods rich in amino acids, dietary fibres associated with complex carbohydrates, and healthy fats and fatty acids. On the contrary, pathogenic bacteria feed upon sugars and refined carbohydrates, and a diet rich in trans fats. In brief, sugars and refined carbohydrates invoke an insulin response from the pancreas every time they enter the body system. Over time, increased insulin levels stimulate the production of pro-inflammatory molecules, contributing to inflammation in the gut lining, resulting in a leaky gut.

Anything else that is fuelling the epidemic of mental illnesses? Yes! In addition to processed food, it is the daily stress we endure and the poor lifestyle choices we make.

Whenever we face a stressful situation—be it chasing a deadline or something as simple as waking up late—our body induces a stress response, ultimately releasing cortisol which is also referred to as the 'stress hormone'. The stress response is a natural reaction to our life experiences. However, sustained psychological stressors such as work-related pressures, relationship difficulties or financial strains can lead to the chronic activation

---

[5]Chen, Y., J. Xu, and Y. Chen, 'Regulation of Neurotransmitters by the Gut Microbiota and Effects on Cognition in Neurological Disorders', *Nutrients*, Vol. 13, No. 6, 2021, https://tinyurl.com/27bm64hd. Accessed on 13 March 2025.

of the stress response. This persistent activation results in the prolonged elevation of cortisol levels, leading to a state of **cortisol dysregulation.** This dysregulation has been associated with various mental health issues over time, including anxiety disorders, depression and cognitive impairments.

What goes on behind being depressed, anxious, or simply apathetic is something that is much greater than what meets the eye. What looks pacific on the surface has a storm looming inside. Pointing fingers at a poor diet and daily stress might seem very convenient, but there is a whole lot of science involved in it. Because of these complexities, it is essential to understand the whys and hows of the progression of mental health symptoms (discussed in Part 1) before we understand 'what' we can do to prevent and treat them, because only then will our solutions (discussed in Part 2) make more sense.

1

The Gut-Brain Axis and Mental Health

Until recent years, medical research studies kept ignoring the significant role played by two of the most complex and critical organ systems of our bodies in maintaining our overall health: the gut (the digestive system) and the brain (the nervous system). The research reflected the idea that the digestive system and the brain were largely independent of each other. However, we now know that the gut and the brain are intricately connected as a bidirectional biochemical signalling network which we call the gut-brain axis.

Now, before we proceed further towards explaining the gut-brain axis, let's first understand what neurotransmitters exactly are and how they are released inside the body. I apologize in advance if it gets a bit too technical, but I will try to explain it in as easy a language as possible. There will be some technical terms you need not remember, but just try to understand how the system works. So let's begin.

Understanding Neurotransmitters and Neurotransmission

Neurotransmitters are chemical messengers that play a crucial role in transmitting signals across the nervous system. They are the key players in the complex communication network of the brain and the body, facilitating everything from basic bodily functions to intricate thoughts and emotions. Neurotransmission—the process by which these neurotransmitters are released and transmit signals between neurons—is fundamental to how we experience, interact with and respond to the world around us.

What Are Neurotransmitters?

Neurotransmitters are chemicals produced by neurons, the specialized cells of the nervous system. These neurotransmitters carry signals from one neuron to another across a tiny gap known as a synapse. They can either excite or inhibit the receiving neuron, depending on the type of neurotransmitter and receptors involved. This process is critical for the functioning of the nervous system, and underlies all neural communication.

Key Functions of Neurotransmitters

Neurotransmitters are involved in a wide range of functions, including:

- **Mood Regulation:** Neurotransmitters like serotonin, dopamine and norepinephrine are crucial in regulating mood and emotional states. An imbalance in these chemicals can lead to mood disorders such as depression and anxiety.
- **Cognitive Functions:** Neurotransmitters such as acetylcholine and glutamate are involved in learning, memory and other cognitive processes.
- **Motor Control:** Neurotransmitters like dopamine play a role in controlling movement and coordination. Deficiencies in dopamine, for instance, are associated with Parkinson's disease.

- **Sleep and Wakefulness:** Neurotransmitters like GABA (gamma-aminobutyric acid) and histamine regulate sleep cycles and alertness.
- **Pain Perception:** Endorphins and other neurotransmitters help modulate pain and can induce feelings of pleasure.

What Is Neurotransmission?

Neurotransmission is the process by which neurotransmitters are released from one neuron and travel across the synapse to transmit signals to another neuron or a target cell. This process is essential for communication within the nervous system, and that between the nervous system and the rest of the body.

The Synthesis of Neurotransmitters: The Role of the Brain, Central Nervous System and Gut

Neurotransmitters are synthesized primarily in the brain and the central nervous system (CNS), but the gut also plays a significant role in their production, highlighting the importance of the gut-brain axis.

- **Brain:** The brain is the primary site for the synthesis of many neurotransmitters. For example, dopamine is synthesized in the substantia nigra and the ventral tegmental area, serotonin is synthesized in the raphe nuclei, and acetylcholine is produced in various regions including the basal forebrain.
- **Central Nervous System (CNS):** Beyond the brain, neurotransmitters are also synthesized in other parts of the CNS including the spinal cord. The CNS is responsible for coordinating the release and action of these neurotransmitters, ensuring that they are available

where needed for the communication between neurons.
- **The Gut:** The gut, often referred to as the 'second brain', is home to the enteric nervous system (ENS), a network of neurons embedded in the lining of the gastrointestinal system. This system is capable of producing neurotransmitters such as serotonin, which is predominantly synthesized in the gut; about 90 per cent of the body's serotonin is found here.
- **The Influence of Gut Microbiota:** The gut microbiota—the trillions of microorganisms living in the digestive tract—also play a critical role in neurotransmitter synthesis. These microbes can produce, modify and influence the levels of neurotransmitters like serotonin, dopamine and GABA. For example, certain gut bacteria can produce short-chain fatty acids (SCFAs) that influence the production of neurotransmitters in the CNS.

Now that we have established the basic role of the brain and the gut in the production of neurotransmitters, let's try to understand how they interact with each other, and further expand on the role of neurotransmitters in affecting our mental health and overall well-being.

The Gut-Brain Axis: A Two-Way Street

The gut-brain axis refers to the constant bidirectional dialogue between the enteric nervous system (ENS) located in the gut, and the central nervous system (CNS) which is primarily the brain. This connection allows the gut to influence brain function and vice versa, playing a crucial role in the regulation of neurotransmitter levels and consequently in our mental health and well-being. This communication occurs through various pathways, including the vagus nerves, neurotransmitters, hormones and immune system molecules. Simply put, signals travel from the gut to the brain and vice versa. For instance:

What happens when we experience butterflies in our stomach? It is the stress or nervousness that is impacting our gastrointestinal functions, leading to symptoms like abdominal discomfort. In extreme cases, stress has been shown to cause diarrhoea or vomiting.

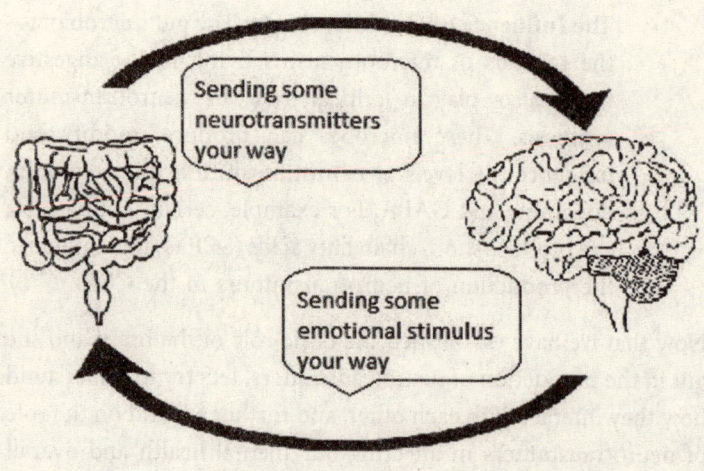

Figure 1: Representation of the gut-brain axis and its bidirectional communication

Conversely, disturbances in gut microbiota composition—known as **gut dysbiosis**—adversely influence brain function and behaviour by downregulating neurotransmitters and producing inflammatory molecules. Located in the gut, the ENS comprises 50–100 million nerve cells—as many as there are in our spinal cord—which empowers the gut to actually outclass all the other organs in terms of functional capabilities, and match the brain's performance.

How Does the Gut Influence Neurotransmission?

- **Neurotransmitter Production:** As mentioned earlier, the gut is a significant site of neurotransmitter production. For instance, the gut microbiota can produce the precursors to neurotransmitters, such as tryptophan for serotonin synthesis.
- **Immune System Interaction:** The gut is a major player in the immune system which can impact neurotransmitter levels and function. Inflammatory responses in the gut can influence the brain, leading to changes in neurotransmitter production and signalling.
- **Vagus Nerve:** The vagus nerve is a key component of the gut-brain axis, providing a direct line of communication between the gut and the brain. It helps transmit signals related to the gut's environment which can affect neurotransmitter production and release.

How Does the Brain Influence the Gut?

- **Stress Response:** The brain's response to stress can influence gut function, leading to changes in the gut motility,[6] gut permeability and neurotransmitter release in the gut.
- **Hormonal Signals:** The brain can send signals through hormones like cortisol that affect the gut's environment and its ability to produce neurotransmitters.

We often see people emphasizing paying attention to one's 'gut feeling' while making decisions or dealing with certain situations.

---

[6] Gut motility refers to the movement of food from the mouth through the pharynx (throat), oesophagus, stomach, small and large intestines, and out of the body.

This expression is not just randomly made up. A healthy gut is considered to make the brain more agile and cognitively enhanced. The gut can influence our emotional responses to pain, happiness, failure or success. It also plays a role in how we interact socially and even guides many of our decisions. When 'Sarah' hung out with her colleagues for dinner or lunch, and attended office parties, it was her decision to project a fancy version of herself in front of her colleagues and on social media. Eventually when she felt lonely and became disappointed, she decided to isolate herself. It was her 'gut feelings' sending wrong signals to the brain, causing her to make poor decisions. Neurotransmitters such as serotonin, dopamine and GABA are primarily synthesized in the gut and exert a profound effect on mood, cognition and behaviour, which is why it's a no-brainer that the gut is often referred to as the 'second brain'.

The gut houses millions of neurons and harbours trillions of microorganisms that regulate digestion, nutrient absorption and immune function, influencing our overall health. Approximately 90 per cent of the body's serotonin—a neurotransmitter involved in regulating mood and appetite—is produced in the gut. Similarly, hormones like cortisol and ghrelin which modulate our stress response and appetite are influenced by gut microbiota activity. Disruptions in this activity have been linked to various physical and mental health conditions including obesity, inflammatory bowel disease, depression and anxiety.

The Mind-Body Connection: Exploring the Intensity of the Gut-Brain Axis

Mounting evidence suggests that disturbances in the gut-brain axis are linked to various psychiatric disorders, including depression, anxiety and autism spectrum disorders. The gut microbiota composition has been found to differ between individuals with mood disorders and healthy controls, highlighting the potential therapeutic implications of targeting gut health in mental health interventions.

However, when we talk about mental health, we use a term that is loosely interchangeable with the brain, the heart, or at times, even the gut. It is the **mind**. The mind, as we know, does not have a physical existence. However, it is integral to the body—the essence of our being. It is the home of our consciousness, including our emotions, feelings, cognition and thoughts, but cannot be confined to just the brain or the gut alone, although it is very well connected to them both.

Simply put, the mind is much more than
what happens in our gut or brain.
However, our gut and brain can definitely shape the mind.

For centuries, the intricate relationship between the mind and the body has fascinated philosophers, scientists and healers alike. From Descartes's dualism to modern neuroscientific discoveries, understanding how our mental and physical states are intertwined has been a pursuit central to human well-being. The mind-body connection is as real as breathing or the beating of our hearts; it is a biological fact that persists whether we realize it or not. It has emerged as an essential link to understanding the body's holistic health, and an integral part of this connection is the gut-brain axis—hardwired as anatomical linkages between the brain and the gut, and facilitated via biological (mainly neurological and psychological) signals carried throughout the bloodstream.

The gut-brain axis is how the mind-body
connection manifests itself physiologically.

While the brain has long been recognized as the primary seat of consciousness and cognition, the gut has emerged as a surprising player in shaping mental processes. Modern research has expanded our understanding of the mind to encompass the intricate interplay and communication pathways between various physiological systems, most importantly the brain and the gut.

Understanding the dynamics of the brain-gut axis is paramount for comprehending the multifaceted nature of the mind and its implications for mental health. By embracing an integrated approach that considers the interconnectedness of body and mind, we can foster holistic well-being and pave the way for a more comprehensive understanding of human cognition and behaviour. Instead of treating symptoms in isolation, addressing underlying gut imbalances can promote comprehensive health outcomes. Lifestyle factors such as diet, stress management, sleep hygiene and probiotic supplementation can positively influence the gut-brain axis, fostering resilience against physical and mental health challenges.

So how exactly does the gut-brain axis modulate mental health? The straight answer is: via neurotransmitters and neurotransmission.

Over the past decades, scientists and medical professionals have understood and confirmed the neurotransmitters' role in the progression of anxiety and depression. Simultaneously, we have also been presented with multiple proofs pointing at the importance of gut microbiota in the pathogenesis of anxiety and depression. Hence, it is not difficult to link an unhealthy gut with inadequate production of neurotransmitters and defective neural signalling, leading to emotional distress.

> Brain neurotransmitter modulation by gut microbiota is indispensable to the pathology of anxiety and depression,[7] with insufficient levels of neurotransmitters (mainly serotonin, dopamine and norepinephrine) being postulated as one of the major factors leading to the latter.

Gut-Derived Neurotransmitters Regulate Mental Health

Central to the gut-brain relationship are neurotransmitters—chemical messengers that facilitate communication between neurons. The gut houses the production and utilization of more than 30 classes of neurotransmitters, which are also identified in the CNS. Gut microbiota alter the levels of neurotransmitters by producing them directly or regulating the related metabolism pathways—something we will keep exploring throughout the book. The imbalance of neurotransmitters is one of the primary reasons for the distress or impairment of personal mental health.

More than 90 per cent of the body's serotonin is synthesized in the gut. Also, the gut produces and stores about 50 per cent of the body's dopamine.

Studies have most often attributed mental disorders to the dysregulation of neurotransmitters like serotonin, dopamine, norepinephrine and GABA.[8] Let's explore such prominent neurotransmitters which are produced in the gut, play the most

---

[7]Huang, F., and X. Wu, 'Brain Neurotransmitter Modulation by Gut Microbiota in Anxiety and Depression', Frontiers in Cell and Developmental Biology, Vol. 9, 649103, 2021, https://tinyurl.com/35wf3kth. Accessed on 13 March 2025.

[8]Liu, T., et al., 'Influence of Gut Microbiota on Mental Health via Neurotransmitters: A Review', Journal of Artificial Intelligence for Medical Sciences, Vol. 1, No. 1–2, 2020, pp. 1–14.

significant roles in promoting mental health and well-being, and are found to act as mediators between gut microbiota and mental disorders.

1. Serotonin—*Natural Mood Regulator*

Serotonin is one of the most important neurotransmitters influencing overall well-being, playing an integral role across various physiological systems. For instance, it helps promote glucose uptake by muscle tissues, thereby regulating blood sugar levels. Also, it is responsible for regulating various gastrointestinal (GI) activities such as the emptying of the stomach, thereby regulating our appetite. Serotonin is made from the essential amino acid tryptophan, which must enter our body through our diet. Tryptophan is commonly found in meat, dairy products, eggs and nuts (details of which you will find in Part 2).

Impact on Mental Health

Serotonin is widely known for its regulatory effect on our mood and is considered to be a natural mood stabilizer. It allows our body to manage anxiety and experience happiness. Additionally, it also plays an important role in:

- Anger management
- Fear perception
- Coping with stress
- Keeping our memory sharpened
- Regulating our appetite
- Addiction
- Experiencing sexual pleasure
- Regulating sleep and wakefulness
- Pain perception

There is substantial evidence linking defects in the metabolism and signalling of serotonin to different psychiatric disorders such as major depressive disorder, anxiety, post-traumatic stress disorder (PTSD), obsessive-compulsive disorder (OCD), eating disorders, schizophrenia, autism and aggressive behaviours. It is the primary therapeutic target when it comes to treating mental health ailments such as major depressive disorder and anxiety disorders. Several drugs (such as SSRIs[9]) targeting serotonin are reasonably effective therapeutic agents in all of these conditions.

2. Dopamine—*Rewards with Pleasure*

It's a game of cards. The cards in your hands don't seem to be good enough, but you still try to figure out a way to manipulate your opponents, and you win right when your best friend thought he was about to beat you! You exclaim in joy, ecstatic with victory. Familiar with the feeling? Or let me take simpler examples of just following a routine—exercising daily at a scheduled time; finishing your work before you planned and realizing that you've earned half an hour for your leisure activities; or getting intimate with your loved one. It's this sort of feeling that gives us happiness, pleasure, satisfaction or a sense of achievement—which dopamine is involved in making us feel. It does so by acting on the areas of the brain responsible for triggering such feelings.

Impact on Mental Health

Dopamine plays an essential role in the brain's reward system, where it reinforces feelings of pleasure that people experience

---

[9] SSRIs: Selective serotonin reuptake inhibitors are the class of drugs that treat depression and anxiety by increasing levels of serotonin in the brain. They do it by blocking the reabsorption (reuptake) of serotonin into neurons, making more serotonin available to improve the transmission of messages between neurons.

when they engage in rewarding activities. Here, the keyword is 'reinforcing', not 'producing'. Just to be clear, dopamine does not produce pleasure but reinforces the feeling thereof by linking that 'joyous' feeling with a certain activity, which arouses the urge to do that activity again. Dopamine also has a role to play in:

- Boosting learning and memory
- Regulating mood
- Staying alert
- Doing a task with focus and concentration
- Staying motivated

> **When the Feel-Good Hormone Goes Bad**
> An increase in dopamine in the brain while achieving something, playing or doing a recreational activity (for example, gambling or taking drugs) can cause you to feel so excited that you might start wanting to feel more of this dopamine 'reward', which is how dopamine plays a role in developing addiction.

A lack of dopamine can prevent a person from feeling pleasure and cause him or her to feel emotionally aloof and withdrawn—which are often also symptoms of clinical depression. Dopamine deficiency can also reduce one's sexual drive and induce forgetfulness, anxiousness and inattentiveness. Decreased effectiveness in dopamine metabolism and signalling can cause symptoms of lethargy, diminished appetite and cravings for sweet or junk food.

3. GABA—*The Calming Messenger*

We are all aware of how proteins are made of amino acids. GABA is also an amino acid, but it is not a part of any protein. It serves as a neurotransmitter well known for inducing calming effects by slowing down or blocking specific signals in the brain. GABA-producing neurons in the gut communicate bidirectionally with the brain, influencing emotional states and stress responses.

Impact on mental health

Due to its ability to induce a calming effect, GABA serves as a natural antidepressant. It plays a crucial role in:

- Calming the neurons in the brain and CNS
- Regulating and stabilizing your mood
- Modulating stress responses by lowering anxiety
- Managing emotional states
- Improving sleep

The dysregulation of gut-derived GABA has been implicated in conditions such as irritable bowel syndrome (IBS), depression, anxiety disorders and manic mood states, highlighting its significance in maintaining mental well-being.

4. Norepinephrine (aka noradrenaline)—*The Stress Hormone*

'Geeta' has been asked to give a big presentation in front of a client coming to the office the day after tomorrow. She will have to work hard on it as the window is extremely narrow. She knows that this client is very important to the company, and she must impress him so they can get a deal out of him. If all goes well, her boss will definitely give her either a raise or a promotion. However, if she botches the presentation, it can be catastrophic for the company and her reputation. Here's the catch—she can refuse to do it and let somebody else take charge. As she gets input from her manager about what she needs to prepare and what they expect, her heart races to start preparing a blueprint in her mind as to how she needs to go about it. She knows it will be the most stressful 48 hours of her life should she accept. She wonders whether she can deliver it in the given time.

These kinds of situations can put somebody on 'flight' mode, while others choose to take up the challenge and 'fight'. One is required to gather every ounce of energy from their body and mind to collect information and decide. These are called 'fight-or-flight' responses, and norepinephrine is a neurotransmitter and stress hormone involved in the body's fight-or-flight response by helping a person stay alert and focused. Another example of this is when you see a snake or a stray dog growling at you. What you do is what you decide in a matter of seconds. Do you run or scare them away?

Norepinephrine is the opposite of GABA. Where GABA works as a calming agent by blocking certain signals in the brain, norepinephrine induces alertness and bursts of energy by upregulating certain signals. While primarily synthesized in the brainstem, it is also produced in sympathetic neurons within the gut. Gut-derived norepinephrine regulates various gastrointestinal functions including motility, blood flow and immune responses.

Impact on Mental Health

Norepinephrine is a neurotransmitter that messages your body to wake up. The dysregulation of gut-derived norepinephrine has been linked to stress-related disorders, highlighting its role in shaping mental health outcomes. Additionally, norepinephrine plays a crucial role in:

- Short-term and working memory
- Staying motivated and energetic throughout the day
- Staying alert and focused
- Modulating stress resilience and emotional arousal

Feeling lazy and unmotivated are often signs of low levels of noradrenaline, symptoms of which are also associated with major depression. Attention-deficit hyperactivity disorder (ADHD) has also been linked to low noradrenaline levels, causing a person difficulties in focusing and concentrating.

5. Acetylcholine (ACh)

Acetylcholine (ACh) plays a role in arousal, thinking, memory and learning. Like norepinephrine, ACh is also an excitatory neurotransmitter, implying that it excites the nerve cell, causing it to 'fire off the message'.

Impact on Mental Health

ACh systems have a crucial role in the regulation of the sleep-waking cycle. Additionally, ACh is involved in:

- Staying attentive
- Releasing adrenaline and norepinephrine from the adrenal glands, helping in exhibiting all the effects similar to those produced by norepinephrine
- Building long-term and working memory—memory formation, consolidation and retrieval
- Increasing motivation

Low blood levels of choline or acetylcholine have been linked to a higher risk of anxiety, ADHD, dementia and Alzheimer's disease (AD).

6. Melatonin

Melatonin is a chemical that affects your sleep patterns and mood. It is produced by the gut and pineal gland. However, the gut produces and stores 400 times more melatonin than the pineal gland. It enhances the immune system in the gut.

Impact on Mental Health

The opposite of norepinephrine, melatonin is a neurotransmitter that messages your body to sleep, helping in the regulation of the sleep-waking cycle. Additionally, melatonin is involved in:

- Alleviating symptoms of depression
- Lowering restlessness

Melatonin supplements are extremely useful in treating insomnia and its related symptoms in mood disorders and ADHD. Also, melatonin has been found to improve the mood in case of seasonal affective disorder (SAD), also known as winter depression. In some studies, it has also been found to be useful in preventing the relapse of psychiatric disorders in patients in remission.

Screen Time and the 'Blue Light' Effect on Melatonin

If you've gone to get your spectacles made, you must have heard the optometrist telling you how good-quality glasses prevent your eyes from getting affected by 'blue light'. He is actually trying to sell you a lens of better quality over an ordinary one which does not reflect back the blue light and lets it reach your retina. This blue light emitted by electronic devices like smartphones, tablets and computers is detrimental to your eye health. But what the optometrist as well as you might not know is that it can also significantly impact your sleep patterns by interfering with the body's natural production of melatonin.

Melatonin—produced by the pineal gland in the brain—is primarily released during the evening and in the nighttime. It plays a crucial role in regulating the sleep-wake cycle, commonly known as the circadian rhythm. Melatonin levels typically rise in the evening, signalling to the body that it's time to prepare for sleep, and they decrease in the morning signalling wakefulness. However, the blue light emitted by electronic screens suppresses the production of melatonin. It is because this light emitted by screens is the same as the one emitted by the sun in abundance during the day, which serves as the cue for our body to remain awake. So when we expose ourselves to screens in the evening, especially near our bedtime, our bodies interpret this artificial light as a signal to stay awake, leading to a delay in the onset of sleep.

Prolonged exposure to blue light in the evening can confuse the body's internal clock and the circadian rhythm which regulates various biological processes including sleep. This confusion can result in difficulties in falling asleep as the body's natural cues for the onset of sleep are disrupted.

But this does not mean that you can use electronic devices for hours wearing these spectacles late at night, as electronic screen time can disrupt sleep by simply overstimulating your brain, which has nothing to do with the extraordinary quality of your spectacles.

Keep in Mind

The mind encompasses a complex interplay between the brain, the gut and their intricate communication pathways. While the brain has long been recognized as the primary seat of consciousness and cognition, the gut emerges as a surprising player in shaping mental processes. The gut-brain axis serves as a vital link in comprehending the mind-body connection and maintaining holistic health. Its intricate communication network underscores the importance of considering gut health in the management and prevention of various physical and mental health conditions. Gut microbiota regulate the gut's enteric nervous system which helps produce and store neurotransmitters that serve as chemical messengers carrying stimulatory or inhibitory messages.

Neurotransmitters are the essential chemical messengers that enable the brain and the body to communicate, regulate emotions, control movements and maintain homeostasis. The process of neurotransmission—which relies on the delicate balance and precise action of these chemicals—is vital for every aspect of human life.

Neurotransmitters like serotonin, dopamine, norepinephrine, GABA, acetylcholine, and others play critical roles in regulating our mood, modulating stress responses and improving cognition, thereby maintaining our mental health. Imbalances or dysregulation of these neurotransmitters in the gut have implications for mental health, and vice versa. Differences in the levels of neurotransmitters and gut microbiota composition between healthy individuals and patients with mental health symptoms highlight the potential therapeutic implications of targeting the gut in mental health interventions.

The synthesis of neurotransmitters in the brain, the CNS and the gut underscores the importance of a holistic approach to mental and physical health. The gut-brain axis plays a pivotal role in this process, highlighting how interconnected our bodily systems are. By understanding and supporting this complex dance of neurotransmitters, we can better manage our mental health, improve our well-being, and appreciate the intricate symphony that governs our lives.

Table: Summarizing the Role of Neurotransmitters Produced inside the Gut in Enhancing Mental Well-Being

Neurotransmitter	Impact on Mental Health
Serotonin	• Works as a natural mood stabilizer by managing anxiety and letting your body experience happiness • Helps in anger management and coping with stress • Regulates appetite • Enables you to experience sexual pleasure • Regulates sleep and wakefulness • Manages fear and pain perception
Dopamine	• Boosts learning and memory • Regulates mood • Helps you stay alert, focused and motivated
GABA	• Works as a natural anti-depressant by calming the neurons in the brain and CNS • Regulates and stabilizes mood • Modulates stress responses by lowering anxiety • Manages emotional states and improves sleep
Norepinephrine	• Builds short-term and working memory • Helps the body stay alert, motivated, energetic and focused • Modulates stress resilience and emotional arousal

| Acetylcholine | - Regulates the sleep-wake cycle by helping the body to stay attentive
- Exhibits all the effects similar to those produced by norepinephrine
- Builds long-term and working memory—memory formation, consolidation and retrieval |
|---|---|
| Melatonin | - Regulates the sleep-wake cycle by messaging the body to sleep
- Lowers restlessness |

2

Understanding Leaky Gut: Why Food for Our Microbiome Matters

There was a time when he was unabashed about how he looked, his eating habits, and where he spent time. 'Manoj', a 29-year-old man, did not think twice before heading to fancy restaurants or partying at a pub late at night and having a few drinks too many. Apart from hanging out with his friends, he had a pretty sedentary lifestyle, leading to obesity.

Without showing an iota of concern, Manoj kept living the same life as he did before becoming obese. Consequently, he developed other symptoms such as bloating, high blood pressure and reflux. When he constantly began feeling lazy, fatigued and less agile, he realized that his health was deteriorating, mainly due to his choices. Upon looking at himself in the mirror, he felt guilty and embarrassed about what he had become. His poor self-image impacted his interpersonal relationships. The identity crisis worsened when he began comparing himself with his friends who were lean, healthier, stronger and smarter. Spiralling downwards, he stopped going out with his friends due to being conscious of his 'fatty' appearance. Furthermore, he reported frequent episodes of emotional eating as a coping mechanism for stress and negative emotions, further exacerbating his weight gain.

Manoj saw a couple of psychiatrists who put him on a cocktail of anti-depressants. He was put on venlafaxine, lithium and mirtazapine to improve depressive symptoms. He was also prescribed admenta and naltrexone to enhance his cognitive functions and help him quit drinking.

Upon examination, Manoj exhibited signs of malnutrition and inflammation, with blood tests indicating micronutrient deficiencies and elevated C-reactive protein (CRP) levels (an inflammation marker). His lactulose and mannitol test was found positive for intestinal permeability. Stool analysis revealed gut dysbiosis characterized by reduced levels of beneficial bacteria and an abundance of opportunistic pathogens. Serum zonulin levels—one of the very few markers of intestinal permeability—were also significantly elevated, confirming the diagnosis of leaky gut syndrome. Furthermore, we conducted hydrogen and methane breath tests, which showed elevated levels of both gases in his breath, further validating gut abnormality.

Zonulin is a protein that plays a role in regulating intestinal permeability. The more zonulin there is in the body, the greater the intestinal permeability and the less the integrity of the gut lining.

A recent study showed the effect of the leaky gut in the progression of depressive disorders through changes in the production of neurotransmitters and other metabolites derived from gut microbiota.[10] It also linked factors like a carbohydrate-rich diet and related dietary habits, psychosocial stress, a sedentary lifestyle, smoking, drinking and antibiotic or painkiller-consumption with poor gut microbiota and the development of depressive disorders.

---

[10]Nohesara, S., et al., 'Microbiota-Induced Epigenetic Alterations in Depressive Disorders Are Targets for Nutritional and Probiotic Therapies', *Genes*, Vol. 14, No. 12, 2217, 2023, https://tinyurl.com/y4xkdk5t. Accessed on 17 March 2025.

Understanding Leaky Gut: Why Food for Our Microbiome Matters

> **The Leaky Gut Test**
> We detect a leaky gut via a simple urine investigation called the lactulose and mannitol test, also known as the intestinal permeability test. It is a simple do-at-home test involving drinking a sugary solution comprising mannitol and lactulose. After drinking the solution, one is supposed to collect one's urine in six-hour intervals and send a sample to the lab. If the sugars are not absorbed into the bloodstream and are found in the urine, it confirms the presence of leaky gut syndrome.

As defined earlier, a leaky gut is a condition characterized by the compromised integrity of the intestinal barrier, allowing the passage of toxins, microbes and undigested food particles into the bloodstream. This phenomenon triggers an immune response, leading to inflammation and contributing to the onset and progression of various chronic diseases and mental health disorders.

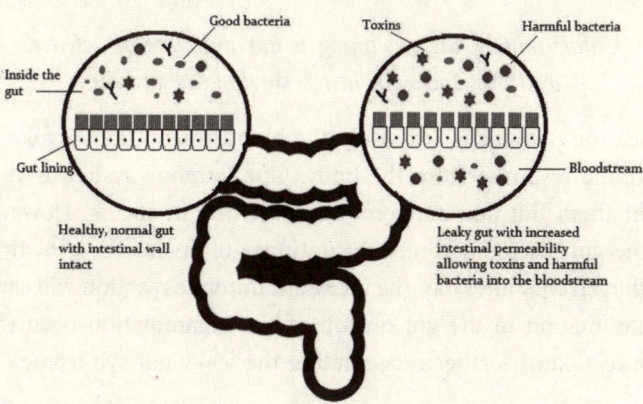

Figure 2: Representation of a normal gut compared to a leaky gut

What Goes on inside the Gut at the Barrier?

The gut lining serves as a barrier separating the bloodstream from pathogens and toxins. The cells of the gut lining are tightly bound to each other like tiles on the floor, but with tiny pores which selectively allow only micronutrients, beneficial metabolites and water into the bloodstream. Inside the gut reside trillions of microbes, both beneficial and pathogenic. Good bacteria play a crucial role in maintaining gut health by either directly producing or facilitating the production of neurotransmitters, metabolites involved in boosting immunity, short-chain fatty acids (SCFAs), and so on. SCFAs, in particular, nourish the cells that line the gut and support a healthy gut barrier.

When the harmful bacteria outnumber the benevolent ones, the amount of toxins and other harmful metabolites increases inside the gut as metabolic byproducts. Overall gut stability is affected, hindering the growth of beneficial bacteria. Consequently, harmful bacteria with their toxic byproducts alter gut permeability and pass through it to enter into the bloodstream.

Unfortunately, the gut lining is our only line of defence, and that too with just a single layer of cells.

Once the pathogens are inside the bloodstream, they invoke an immune response from the body. Our immune system tries to fight them out and suppress any potential ill-effects. However, if the gut microenvironment continues to favour the growth of pathogens day after day, the incessant immune reaction will cause inflammation in the gut on top of the inflammation occurring due to toxins, further exacerbating the leaky gut syndrome.

The overgrowth of pathogenic bacteria overwhelms the number of good bacteria
↓
Good bacteria get crowded out from the gut
↓
It causes an alteration in gut permeability
↓
Pathogenic bacteria, along with their toxic byproducts and unwanted molecules, pass through the gut lining to enter the bloodstream (in a condition known as *leaky gut*)
↓
The body generates an immune response
↓
Inflammation occurs through the gut lining and intestinal wall
↓
The leaky gut worsens

What Causes Pathogenic Bacteria to Overgrow inside the Gut?

Primarily, our eating habits substantially influence the range of gut microbes that thrive in our guts. Health behaviours (eating, smoking, drinking) and environmental factors (exposure to mental stressors and chemicals) have a greater effect on microbiota variability than host genetics. Of all the gut microbes, bacteria are most often studied in matters related to human stress, mood and diet. Poor food choices, a high-stress lifestyle, and many modern practices such as the excessive use of antibiotics, antacids or painkillers promote gut dysbiosis and the low diversity of beneficial bacterial species. Dysbiosis and low diversity alter food cravings, metabolism, stress reactivity and mood—compromising our immune function and health.

Dysbiosis+Low Diversity→A Health Disaster

The recipe for a disaster is as follows:

1. Prepare a base of a sugar-rich diet with processed foods.
2. Spread on top of it some stress, sedentary lifestyle and smoking and drinking sauces.
3. Put some chopped antibiotics and painkillers (narcotics or opioids).
4. Sprinkle some more unhygienic food lacking micronutrients.
5. Now, keep it in the oven for a while, exposing it to different pathogenic bacteria and parasites.

And your leaky gut is ready!

Remember, the base is poor diet and our food choices. But disaster can occur from being exposed to any of the above factors. Even if you do away with the stress sauce and antibiotics, your food choices are enough to promote the growth of harmful bacteria inside the gut and cause leaky gut syndrome.

Tell me what you eat and I will tell you who you are.

—Jean Anthelme Brillat-Savarin, French gastronome

A healthy diet can help you cope with the stress you endure on a day-to-day basis. It can also alleviate the negative effects of the cocktail of medications you take. However, you cannot out-medicate an unhealthy diet. Even if you exercise, meditate, or don't take much stress, you cannot outrun an unhealthy diet.

A 'SAD' Diet—Something Our Gut Hates Having

Since we are focusing on those aspects of gut functioning that affect mental health, the acronym given for the standard American diet, 'SAD', seems more appropriate than ever. However, it is not limited to America. This type of diet has spread all over the globe like an epidemic. With some facets thereof being inculcated in European cuisine, SAD has even corrupted the Mediterranean diet, and has become an integral part of Indian, Chinese and Japanese cuisine. It is characterized by high amounts of processed foods, added sugars, and refined carbohydrates and fats. It should be no surprise that SAD is also typically low in a variety of healthy and minimally processed foods including vegetables, fruits, legumes and whole grains.

India leads the list of the top 10 countries in the world in terms of the highest number of people with diabetes, followed by China, USA, Russia, Germany and Japan. Hence, in some ways, the standard American diet has become the standard Asian diet, and it is 'sad'.

What Is in Our Diet That Causes It to Become SAD?

Simple as it is, foods rich in refined sugars, simple carbohydrates (for example, fructose and glucose), refined oils and trans fats constitute SAD; it kills the growth of beneficial bacteria and empowers pathogens to overgrow. Additionally, food products low in fibre can cause dysregulation of the immune function, which further affects our gut health.

> *Some pathogens are so sensitive that they overgrow within 24 hours of eating junk food.*

Let's look at these food categories one by one:

1. Refined sugars, fructose or high-fructose corn syrup

Examples: table sugars, candies, cookies, soft drinks, aerated drinks and fruits like grapes, dates, figs, mangoes, lychees, and so on. Sugars serve as food for pathogenic bacterial species such as the *Streptococcus* bacteria. The persistent intake of sugars like glucose and fructose results in the overcrowding of harmful bacteria, leading to a leaky gut. Also, they spike insulin levels which, after a point, invoke an inflammatory response further damaging the gut lining.

2. Products containing refined carbohydrates

Examples: white flour, white rice, cereals, pastries, sodas, pizza, pasta, white bread, buns and burgers, bakery sweets, and so on. They break down into glucose fairly quickly, contributing to a persistent state of hyperglycaemia, generating the same inflammatory response as stated above, and damaging the gut lining and causing the gut to leak.

3. Vegetable oils (processed refined oils)

Examples: refined sunflower oil, soybean oil, rice bran oil, corn oil, cottonseed oil, sesame oil, *dalda, vanaspati,* and so on. These oils have high amounts of omega-6 fatty acids which multiple studies have linked to the pathogenesis of many disorders, including cancer, cardiovascular disease and inflammatory diseases.[11] Generally, omega-6 fatty acids are allowed to be consumed in limited quantities. The advised ratio of consuming omega-6 and omega-3 fatty acids is 4:1 to 6:1, which means that for every 1 gram of omega-3, one can consume up to 4 to 6 grams of omega-6. However, our SAD diet, typically containing fried foods, now offers omega-6 and 3 in the ratio of 20:1.

---

[11] DiNicolantonio, J.J., and J. O'Keefe, 'The Importance of Maintaining a Low Omega-6/Omega-3 Ratio for Reducing the Risk of Autoimmune Diseases, Asthma, and Allergies', *Missouri medicine*, Vol. 118, No. 5, 2021, https://tinyurl.com/ya66dhur. Accessed on 17 March 2025.

Omega-3 and omega-6 are polyunsaturated essential fatty acids (PUFA). Without going into the science of poly-, mono- and unsaturated fatty acids, all we need to note is that **omega-6** and **omega-3** are **essential** for our body, implying that our body cannot synthesize them on its own and they must be consumed by us in the form of food. While omega-3 has consistently been shown to lead to positive outcomes in health, large amounts of omega-6 have been linked to inflammation, cancer and cardiovascular diseases. Studies have shown that when taken in the ratio of 2:1 to 5:1, these fatty acids, in combination, suppress inflammation and reduce the risk of cancer and cardiovascular disorders.[12]

Does Omega-6 Also Play a Role in Causing a Leaky Gut?

Yes! The link lies in its interaction with HNF-4 alpha, a protein responsible for maintaining the integrity of the gut lining. When large amounts of omega-6 bind to HNF-4 alpha, they disrupt its functioning thereby weakening the intestinal barrier and causing the gut to leak. A limited intake of omega-6 ensures that it is used elsewhere in other metabolic pathways. But large amounts of omega-6 accumulate inside the gut and interfere in the functioning of HNF-4 alpha.

Refined vegetable oils like soybean and rice bran oils upset the omega-3-to-omega-6 fatty acids ratio inside the gut. Omega-3, to exhibit its health benefits, must be metabolized into anti-inflammatory byproducts by certain beneficial enzymes. When the gut environment is swamped with omega-6, it

---

[12]Simopoulos, A.P., 'The importance of the ratio of omega-6/omega-3 essential fatty acids', *Biomed Pharmacother*, Vol. 56, No. 8, 2002, https://tinyurl.com/59pbfruf. Accessed on 17 March 2025.

depletes these enzymes in the organ, leading to a decrease in anti-inflammatory molecules. Furthermore, pro-inflammatory molecules overgrow, killing helpful bacteria such as the probiotic *Lactobacillus* species.

> ### The Dopamine Connection to Processed Foods
>
> Dopamine, as previously discussed, is a chemical messenger in the brain that plays a crucial role in various functions central to motivation, reward and pleasure. When we eat foods high in sugar, trans fats and salt—common characteristics of processed foods—our brain's reward system is activated, stimulating dopamine release. This is because the brain is wired to seek out pleasurable experiences and processed foods are often engineered to be highly palatable, meaning they stimulate our taste buds and trigger a strong dopamine response. Now the release of dopamine reinforces behaviours resulting in pleasure and satisfaction, making processed foods particularly appealing as they invoke those very feelings when consumed. This intense dopamine response, also referred to as the 'dopamine rush', can lead to cravings and overeating, and cause the mind to seek these types of food repeatedly.
>
> The issue gets more critical when this pleasure-seeking behaviour becomes excessive or uncontrollable. Over time, repeated exposure to highly palatable processed foods can lead to the desensitization of the brain's reward system, stimulating the need to consume larger quantities or more intense flavours to experience the same level of pleasure. As a result, individuals may find themselves eating larger portions of processed foods without feeling satisfied, which, as a result, contributes to overeating and potential weight gain. Furthermore, the rapid

> spike and subsequent drop in blood sugar levels caused by processed foods can exacerbate cravings and contribute to a cycle of overeating and poor dietary choices.

4. Products Containing Trans Fats

Examples: processed butter, potato chips, hamburgers, french fries, popcorn, frozen chicken products, cakes and crackers, cookies and biscuits, doughnuts, and so on. Trans fats are artificial fatty acids produced in the food production process. These fatty acids alter the gut microbiota in favour of pathogenic bacteria, causing gut dysbiosis. By doing so, they also suppress the growth of beneficial microbes responsible for shaping the immune response and producing metabolites involved in maintaining normal physiology.

5. Alcohols

Examples: whiskey, scotch, brandy, vodka, tequila, and such others. Similar to consuming products containing trans fats, moderate-to-heavy alcohol consumption directly alters the biodiversity of gut microbes, producing dramatic changes in the relative abundance of some particular microbes, and causing dysbiosis and inflammation in the gut. *Remember our friend HNF-4 alpha?* Ethanol, the main component of every kind of alcoholic drink, has been found to suppress its expression, causing the gut lining to become leaky.

Protein Putrefaction—A Hidden Phenomenon

Another phenomenon triggered by unhealthy foods affecting gut health is putrefaction. In simple terms, putrefaction is an anaerobic process[13] of protein breakdown. Putrefaction inside the gut refers to the decomposition or fermentation of undigested proteins by the organ's microbiota. The undigested proteins are broken down into amino acids in the large intestine, which are then metabolized by certain harmful bacteria, producing toxic byproducts. When produced excessively, these harmful byproducts like ammonia, amines, phenol, and others are proven to be detrimental to gut health. Previous research has suggested that these toxic metabolites play a significant part in the development of gastrointestinal disorders.[14]

Additionally, when pathogenic bacteria ferment amino acids like tyrosine, they render them unavailable to facilitate neurotransmitter production, mimicking dietary depletion. Contrary to protein decomposition producing toxic byproducts, the fermentation of complex carbohydrates helps maintain stability in the gut environment and integrity of the gut lining *(which we will discuss in detail later in Part 2).*

The foul smell in your breath may be because of excessive protein putrefaction in your gut.

It's not that putrefaction does not occur upon eating healthier foods. It does, but in a limited manner. Excessive putrefaction can only occur if pathogens are outnumbering probiotics. And that happens when we feed our gut the SAD diet with excessive refined oils, omega-6, refined carbohydrates, sugars, alcohol and trans fats.

---

[13] Anaerobic process: It is the bacterial breakdown of organic materials in the absence of oxygen.

[14] Hughes, R., E.A. Magee, and S. Bingham, 'Protein degradation in the large intestine: relevance to colorectal cancer', *Current Issues in Intestinal Microbiology*, Vol. 1, No. 2, 2000, pp. 51–58, https://tinyurl.com/3v36nhyf. Accessed on 17 March 2025.

Eating Habits that Cause Excessive Putrefaction

It is worth noting that proteins need an absolutely acidic environment in the stomach for their digestion. On the contrary, an alkaline environment is required for starch to get digested and absorbed. Hence, when we eat protein-rich food along with starch-rich food, it increases the amount of undigested food because our stomach cannot be acidic and alkaline at the same time. More often than not, our eating habits make our stomach and gut environment neutral to alkaline. Hence, it is more often the protein that remains undigested and gets attacked by pathogenic bacteria, causing protein putrefaction.

> ### Eating Habits That Make Your Stomach Alkaline
>
> Due to there being less acid in the stomach, enzymes like pepsin, trypsin and chymotrypsin cannot digest protein as they need an acidic environment with a pH of 1–3. The following are some of our eating habits that deprive protein-digesting enzymes of the acidic environment they need:
> - Eating fried rice with cooked pulses
> - Drinking water while or immediately after eating food
> - Drinking liquid, be it water, tea or juice after eating
> - Eating eggs with bread—hence, bread-omelette is a big no-no!
> - Eating rapidly and not chewing the food properly—does not allow amylase, an enzyme present in the saliva, to get mixed with the food and digest starch, which means that the stomach has to put in extra effort making the environment alkaline
>
> Of note, our oral cavity, by default, is alkaline. Starch digestion begins from the mouth. However, protein digestion begins only

> inside the stomach. Hence, we must do everything we can to promote an acidic environment inside the stomach. Else, when undigested protein reaches the gut, it will undergo putrefaction.

So What Happens if We Cannot Keep Our Stomach Acidic?

You know it—professionals call it reflux, but the phenomenon is more popularly named acidity, albeit 'acidity' is something we require inside the gut. However, the inability of our GI system to digest food in a less acidic environment pushes the food back up the digestive tract. This is because low stomach acid levels cause the food in the stomach to sit longer to get digested. As the stomach pushes the food back up into the unprotected tissues of the oesophagus, some amount of acid produced by the stomach also gets out into the digestive tract, causing symptoms such as sour burps and heartburn. That's why antacids are not a great option when suffering from reflux, as the symptoms occur only when the gut and stomach are less acidic. Antacids only make the condition worse.

When a patient comes to me with persistent symptoms of reflux, I put them on a combination of probiotics and pepsin and betaine HCL supplement. Probiotics help rejuvenate the gut with beneficial bacteria. On the other hand, betaine HCl increases stomach acid, allowing the pepsin enzyme to work and break protein into smaller chains of amino acids that can then be absorbed and used in different metabolic pathways.

Food Is Not the Only Food We Put In Our Gut

Health is what we strive for—something that we consciously put effort into so that we can remain agile, sharp and fit. Nobody likes being sick. So when we get down with infectious symptoms or experience pain, we first go to a pharmacist and get an antibiotic or a painkiller without even bothering to know if we have a bacterial or a viral infection, without bothering to deduce whether the pain is muscular or originating from our nerves, and certainly without looking for alternative treatment options like drinking herbal tea in case of infections, or applying heat or getting a massage for pain management. Worse still, we do not go to a physician. This is especially true in the context of healthcare in India and other developing countries.

> *What we do not realize is that we are treating our sickness at the cost of our health.*

I say this because we usually do not consult our general physicians to get a confirmed diagnosis. We take antibiotics in case of a viral infection, ending up killing probiotic bacteria that were supposed to fight the infection. We take so much pain medication that our natural tolerance to pain decreases to the extent that we can no longer move without taking a painkiller. Along with antacids, antibiotics and analgesics are the two classes of drugs that are most commonly used in the wrong manner, which eventually causes more harm than good.

The Case of Indiscriminate Action by Antibiotics

Most antibiotics act on a broad spectrum of bacterial species without discriminating between beneficial bacteria and pathogens. Along with killing harmful pathogens, they also end up killing or inhibiting the growth of probiotics. When antibiotics are administered, they can disrupt the delicate balance of gut microbiota, leading to dysbiosis. The overgrowth of harmful bacteria and the depletion of beneficial ones compromise the integrity of the intestinal lining, making it more permeable.

Simply put, antibiotics can disturb the balance of the intestinal microbiome, potentially exacerbating leaky gut syndrome.

Moreover, some antibiotics have been found to directly damage the gut lining by disrupting the tight junctions between intestinal epithelial cells. This disruption allows toxins, undigested food particles and harmful bacteria to pass through the intestinal barrier and enter the bloodstream, triggering inflammation and immune responses.

Painkillers—Used as Gut Killers?

There are two major groups of painkillers: anti-inflammatory analgesics and opioids (aka narcotics). The most common analgesics are NSAIDs (nonsteroidal anti-inflammatory drugs) such as ibuprofen, naproxen and aspirin. They are used to alleviate acute pain and reduce inflammation. They work by inhibiting the activity of enzymes that are involved in the production of inflammatory molecules. However, while doing so, they also interfere in the production of those protective molecules that promote the integrity of the gut lining. As a result, long-term use of NSAIDs leads to the erosion of the gut lining and an increased risk of developing conditions such as peptic ulcers and leaky gut syndrome.

Less commonly used are narcotics that are prescribed for managing chronic and/or severe pain. Their chronic use disrupts how the food particles move in and out of the stomach and the gut, and alters gut microbiota composition, leading to dysbiosis and resulting in increased intestinal permeability. Disruption in the movement of food particles reduces bowel movement frequency, causing constipation, which is a common side effect of using a narcotic. Chronic constipation associated with narcotic use further promotes dysbiosis, exacerbating the issue of leaky gut syndrome.

Furthermore, opioids have been shown to affect gut immune function and intestinal barrier integrity directly. Research suggests that opioids may induce inflammation in the gut mucosa and alter the expression of tight junction proteins essential for maintaining the gut barrier integrity.

In addition to their direct effects on the gastrointestinal tract, narcotics can also indirectly contribute to leaky gut syndrome through their impact on immune function and systemic inflammation. Chronic opioid use has been associated with immune suppression and dysregulation, which can further compromise gut health and contribute to increased intestinal permeability.

Extending what we have already established, this is where we stand in our understanding as of now:

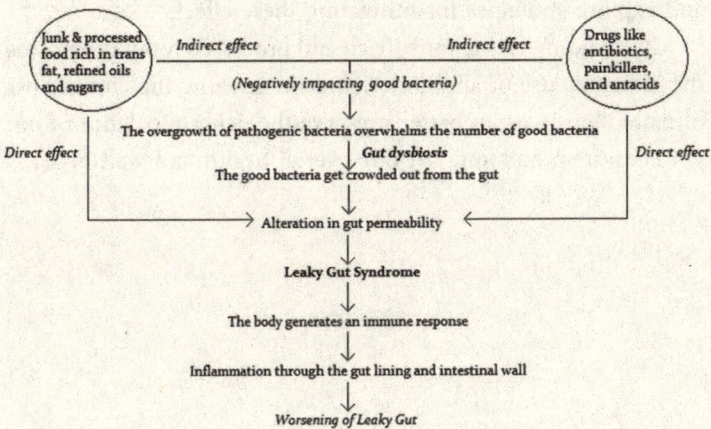

Keep in Mind

'Our health begins from our gut', and we must 'fix the food first' before opting for an extensive exercise regime or expensive clinical intervention. Junk food and processed foods are high in carbohydrates, sugars, trans fats and refined vegetable oils, which we must get rid of. Remember, pathogens feed on sugars and trans fats, whereas probiotics feed on fibre, proteins, micronutrients and other dietary constituents, which we will discuss later in the book.

Antibiotics and painkillers are essential medications in emergencies and cases of trauma; they have revolutionized modern medicine and improved countless lives. However, the prolonged or excessive use thereof in cases of daily discomfort and minor pains has lead people to experience its unintended consequences on gut health, including the development of leaky gut syndrome. As our understanding of the gut microbiota and their role in health and disease continues to evolve, it is crucial to consider the potential impacts of medication on gut health and explore strategies for mitigating these effects.

By avoiding eating junk, fried and processed food, promoting the judicious use of antibiotics, and minimizing the chronic use of painkillers, we can better preserve the delicate balance of our gut ecosystem and support our overall health and well-being.

3

Stress and the Gut: How Our Environment Affects Our Microbiome

When a 35-year-old marketing manager comes to you with complaints of abdominal discomfort, bloating, irregular bowel movements and fatigue, you already know the root cause of her symptoms, especially when she emphasizes how much she loves her job and how happy she is about the way her career is progressing. But the root cause—stress—would always be inevitable in a competitive corporate environment. 'Emma' reported experiencing high levels of stress due to family responsibilities and recent personal challenges. The job was her only escape. However, she always had some deadline or the other to chase, or a critical project to manage.

While explaining her symptoms, Emma mentioned suffering from digestive issues, mild heartburn, and occasional constipation. She led a busy lifestyle, often relying on fast food and caffeine to cope with work demands. She admitted to feeling overwhelmed and anxious, especially during periods of increased stress.

During our initial consultation, Emma appeared tense and worn out. Although her vital signs were within normal limits, she exhibited tenderness upon palpation of the abdomen. This, combined with her reported symptoms, prompted me to order a series of laboratory tests. The results revealed elevated levels of inflammatory biomarkers, including **C-reactive protein (CRP)**[15], and a slightly elevated white blood cell count—both indicative of underlying inflammation. Most telling, however, were the results of her lactulose and mannitol test, which came back positive for intestinal permeability. Elevated serum zonulin levels further confirmed this diagnosis of leaky gut syndrome.

Stress is a natural physiological response to adversity and a significant facet of the body's protection mechanism. Stress can be useful in tiny doses, helping to boost attention, alertness and performance. Chronic stress, on the other hand, can have a toxic influence on multiple body systems, including the gut.

Stressing Our Gut into Leaking

The gut persistently and openly communicates with the brain through the gut-brain axis. When we experience unpleasant situations firsthand, the negative emotions and accompanying stress can perturb gut motility. The gut-brain axis is relevant not only to these transient states, but also to longer-lasting conditions. Digestive disorders such as irritable bowel syndrome commonly coincide with mood disorders including anxiety. These types of disorders may reflect a dysfunctional composition of gut bacteria, viruses and fungi (the gut microbiota), and related chronic inflammation.

Independently and mutually, diet, stress and mood can substantially influence which gut microbes thrive. Many modern

---

[15]CRP: It is a substance produced by the liver in response to inflammation. When CRP levels are elevated, it typically indicates that there is inflammation occurring somewhere in the body. In clinical practice, CRP is often used as a non-specific marker of inflammation to aid in diagnosis, assess disease activity, and monitor response to treatment.

practices such as antibiotic use, a diet rich in carbs, refined vegetable oils and sugars, and high-stress lifestyles promote gut bacterial imbalances as well as low diversity.[16] It is all the more reason why manipulating the gut microbiota and their functions via probiotics and other health behaviours is a promising therapeutic strategy (*which we will discuss later in Part 2*). In the previous chapter, we highlighted the role of poor diet and the indiscriminate use of antibiotics and narcotics in damaging our gut health. Now we take a look at how stress can do the same.

Altering Gut Microbiota Composition

Stress affects our overall well-being through its impact on gut bacteria. With a part of the nervous system working as their playing field, the immune cells serve as biochemical messengers conveying psychological stress to the gut. The heightened inflammation induced by stress triggers the overgrowth of pathogenic bacteria, which thereby encourage dysbiosis and result in a leaky gut.

Affecting Gut Permeability

Stress can induce a lot of behavioural and physiological changes. Behavioural changes include dysregulated eating, having a lot of carb-rich junk food, drinking alcohol, leading a sedentary lifestyle, experiencing altered sleep patterns, and so on. On the other hand, physiological changes include altered immune function. These adverse changes promote the survival and replication of pathogenic gut bacteria, and weaken the gut barrier. These alterations in our behaviour and physiology eventually

---

[16] Low gut microbiota diversity: It refers to a smaller count and uneven distribution of bacterial species inside the gut.

dysregulate key stress-responsive systems, including the immune, endocrine and autonomic nervous systems, thereby fuelling the chronicity of depression and stress.[17]

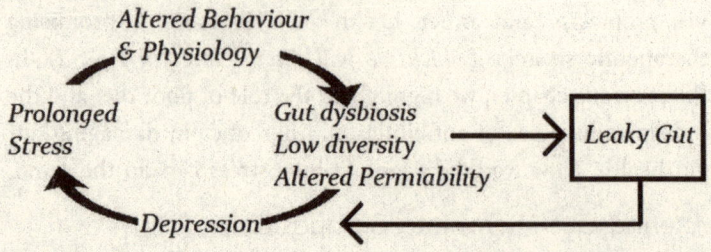

Suppressing the Production of Neurotransmitters

Stress can affect the production of serotonin and GABA, which are crucial to mood and anxiety regulation. As discussed earlier in Chapter 1, these neurotransmitters are produced in the gut by beneficial bacteria. When stress alters the body's physiology, it also lowers gut microbiota diversity to an unfavourable proportion, thereby compromising the production of neurotransmitters, leading to mood disorders.

Impacting Digestive Function

Stress activates the sympathetic nervous system, triggering the body's fight-or-flight response. This response can divert blood flow away from the digestive system, impairing digestion and nutrient absorption. When stress takes a chronic form, it causes certain GI symptoms to develop, such as abdominal pain, bloating

---

[17] Madison, A., and J.K. Kiecolt-Glaser, 'Stress, depression, diet, and the gut microbiota: human-bacteria interactions at the core of psychoneuroimmunology and nutrition', *Current Opinion in Behavioral Sciences*, Vol. 28, 2019, pp. 105–10, https://tinyurl.com/2s43hz3b. Accessed on 18 March 2025.

and irregular bowel movements. When the digestive system is impaired, the small intestine does not get enough nutrients to absorb; whatever it does get access to, it cannot absorb them efficiently. Consequently, the microenvironment inside the gut lining gets drained of nutrients, which hampers the growth of good bacteria, leading to low diversity and gut dysbiosis, and eventually causing a leaky gut.

Compromising the Immune System

As discussed earlier, the gut houses a significant portion of the body's immune system. Gut microbiota—a critical regulator in tuning the mucosal immune system—are essential to the development and functioning of the immune system. However, by altering gut microbiota composition, chronic stress can suppress immune function, making the gut more susceptible to infections and inflammation. This immune dysregulation then contributes to the development or exacerbation of gut-related conditions.

The connection between gut microbiota and stress is bidirectional—stress affects microbiota composition, and the gut microbiome can influence the impact of stress.

Increasing Inflammation and Disrupting the Gut-Brain Axis

As stated earlier, gut-brain communication occurs through various pathways, including the vagus nerve system and others. Here, consider the vagus nerves as brakes which are applied when our brain perceives stress and activates major stress response pathways. By applying the brakes, the gut's nervous system (ENS) reduces intestinal inflammation and strengthens intestinal barrier functions.

The activation of stress response pathways unfolds via the release of adrenaline and noradrenaline. Additionally, stress promotes the release of pro-inflammatory cytokines. Consider these the accelerators of inflammation. Prolonged exposure to stress causes the brakes to fail, allowing inflammation in the gut to continue unchecked. As the brakes fail, stress-induced inflammation turns chronic, compromising intestinal barrier integrity and disrupting gut-brain communication by suppressing the production of neurotransmitters from the gut through the brain.

His Gut Was off and So Was His Mood

This 32-year-old man was otherwise healthy before he started experiencing symptoms of persistent fatigue, bad moods, and decreased interest in activities he used to enjoy. Additionally, he reported difficulty concentrating at work and feeling irritable for no apparent reason. But here was the catch—he also developed GI issues, the timing of which coincided with the mental health symptoms. He described experiencing frequent stomach pain, bloating and occasional nausea, which had been ongoing for several months.

Given the co-occurrence of gastrointestinal symptoms with his mood disturbances, we decided to investigate further for potential underlying causes. His blood test revealed anaemia (low blood count) and elevated inflammatory markers. A stool test for *H. pylori* came back positive with blood in the sample, confirming the presence of the bacterium in his gastrointestinal tract. Apparently, he was bleeding from somewhere internally. Further tests, including an upper endoscopy, confirmed gastritis with bleeding ulcers and the presence of *H. pylori* bacteria in the stomach lining.

The patient, under diligent professional supervision, was put on a combination of antibiotics and a proton pump inhibitor (PPI)[18] for two weeks to eradicate the *H. pylori* infection. Additionally, he was given iron supplements to address his anaemia. To our surprise, before we could address his mental health symptoms directly, he had already begun showing improvements in terms of his mood. He described feeling more relaxed at work and significantly less irritable overall. As the treatment continued with micronutrient supplements and a diet rich in healthy fats, vitamins and foods boosting the production of neurotransmitters, his symptoms—fatigue and bad mood—resolved within four weeks of treating the *H. pylori* infection. Basically, we addressed his mental health issues by treating a GI infection.

Understanding a Different Kind of Threat

The ecosystem of the gut microbiota varies across individuals. Depending on our living environment, dietary habits and drug usage, the structure and function of the microbiota change constantly. We expose our bodies to not only psychosocial stressors every day, but also poor-quality food and polluted environments, allowing pathogens like parasites and worms to enter and colonize the gut. These pathogens then promote gut dysbiosis by triggering the production of inflammatory molecules and causing imbalances in immunity, and the rest we all know.

Small Intestinal Bacterial Overgrowth (SIBO)

As the name suggests, it is a phenomenon where the small intestine is excessively colonized by bacteria that typically grow

---

[18]Proton pump inhibitors (PPIs): Medicines that work by reducing the amount of stomach acid made by glands in the lining of your stomach.

in the large intestine. Normally, the small intestine contains a relatively small number of bacteria. This is because the secretion of gastric acids and intestinal motility limit bacterial growth in the small intestine. Conversely, the failure of these protective mechanisms against excessive bacterial growth translates into small intestinal bacterial overgrowth (SIBO).

The bacterial migration from the colon (large intestine) to the small intestine is a critical factor in the onset and progression of SIBO.

Bacterial migration disrupts the normal digestion process and absorption of nutrients, resulting in bloating, abdominal pain, diarrhoea and malnutrition. The small intestine is lined with tiny finger-like projections called villi which serve as a playing field for nutrient absorption. However, when SIBO occurs, the excessive bacteria present in the small intestine damage these villi, impairing nutrient absorption.

Common Symptoms of SIBO

- Bloating, abdominal pain, diarrhoea or constipation
- Malabsorption of nutrients
- Fatigue and weakness

Bloating or production of excessive gas occurs due to excessive fermentation of carbohydrates and undigested protein (protein putrefaction, as discussed earlier) by abnormally large amounts of bacteria in the small intestine.

The malabsorption of nutrients drains the body of the essential vitamins and minerals it requires to function effectively, further causing impaired immunity, fatigue and lethargy.

When excessive bacteria invade the small intestine, they invoke

> an inflammatory response from the gut, and the same story repeats.
> *Release of pro-inflammatory molecules → Immune response*
> *Persistent invoking of the immune system → Systemic inflammation in the gut*
> ↓
> *Gut dysbiosis*

Impaired intestinal motility is one of the major reasons for the development of SIBO as it causes food to move sluggishly through the GI tract. This sluggish movement of food and waste allows bacteria to linger in the small intestine for longer periods, increasing the risk of overgrowth.

And why would the gut or intestinal motility be affected, you ask? *It is the same old answer—poor diet and psychosocial stress, as we discussed earlier.*

SIBO is different from pathogenic infections in the sense that infections from parasites or worms occur due to ingesting contaminated food or water. However, SIBO occurs due to the excessive growth of bacteria that have already inhabited the digestive tract. Their treatments also require different approaches. Where parasitic infection is treated with anti-parasitic medication, managing SIBO requires a multi-faceted approach involving:

- Dietary control: Following a low FODMAP diet and avoiding fibre-rich and carbohydrate-rich foods
- Lifestyle modifications: Stress management, regular exercise and adequate sleep
- Antibiotics

A Brief Note on Understanding FODMAP

FODMAP stands for fermentable oligosaccharides, disaccharides, monosaccharides and polyols.

To keep it simple, saccharide is a scientific term for sugars and polyols refer to sugar alcohols found in certain fruits, vegetables and artificial sweeteners.

A low FODMAP diet restricts certain carbohydrates, but this isn't the typical low-carb diet. It only eliminates high FODMAP foods and can be individualized, so you only restrict those that trigger your symptoms. Finding the foods that trigger your symptoms typically follows a three-step process.

1. **Elimination:** It involves eliminating all high FODMAP foods for several weeks; symptoms may improve immediately or over several weeks.
2. **Reintroduction:** It involves reintroducing eliminated foods one at a time; identify what you can and cannot tolerate and in what amount.
3. **Personalization:** It involves modification of your dietary habits for the long term depending upon what you've learnt during the reintroduction phase.

Table: Managing SIBO through Dietary Intervention

Foods Allowed ✓	Foods to Avoid ×
Meat, fish, eggs, hard chicken, cheese, tofu and lactose-free yogurt	Sausages, processed meat, breaded meat and cottage cheese
Coconut oil, *desi ghee* and butter	All types of refined vegetable oils like sunflower oil, canola oil, soybean oil and others

Carrots, lettuce, cucumber, pumpkin, quinoa, bean sprouts, eggplant and turnips	Beans, chickpeas, lentils, broccoli and asparagus
Ginger, olives and spring onions	Onions and garlic
Oatmeal and unsweetened cereals	Wheat, gluten-based bread, muffins and biscuits
Fruits like blueberries, raspberries, strawberries, pineapple, grapes and kiwis	Fruits like apples, peaches, pears, mangoes, cherries, figs and dates
Peanuts and walnuts	Almonds, cashews and pistachios

If you notice the table above, the 'to avoid' category contains the list of foods that we would otherwise consider healthy. A low FODMAP diet is not a long-term ritual to follow. Instead, it is a temporary approach to help manage symptoms while identifying specific FODMAP triggers like irritable bowel, bloating, fatigue, persistent constipation, excessive gas, and so on. The spectrum of foods to eat and avoid is very broad when it comes to following a low FODMAP diet. It will become extremely challenging for you to eliminate all the foods in one go. Additionally, you won't know which food to reintroduce first and how. That is why you must follow up with your nutritionist to help you tailor your diet to avoid or limit specific foods while still meeting your nutritional goals. Your nutritionist can help you move forward with your gut-friendly diet, answering questions and sharing low-FODMAP recipes.

Keep in Mind

A healthy gut has a diverse population of bacteria in favour of probiotics. Dysbiosis and low diversity may alter food cravings, metabolism, stress reactivity and mood, compromising your immune function and health. Stress directly induces multiple behavioural and physiological changes, leading to alterations in gut motility, gut diversity and secretion of digestive enzymes. Where low gut motility impacts digestive function, poor diversity suppresses immune function, consequently promoting the development of pro-inflammatory molecules, causing inflammation in the gut. Furthermore, persistent stress affects the availability of neurotransmitters like serotonin, GABA and dopamine, leading to systemic inflammation with further consequences for the gut and brain health. This dysregulation may contribute to symptoms of gastrointestinal disorders and exacerbate stress-related conditions like anxiety and depression.

Stress is not the only stressor we expose our bodies to. Poor-quality food, contaminated water and a polluted environment allow pathogens like parasites and worms to enter and colonize the gut. These pathogens then invoke an inflammatory response and promote gut dysbiosis. On the other hand, SIBO is not a parasitic infection but a case of excessive growth of colonic bacteria in the small intestine. Understanding the science behind SIBO can help individuals seek proper diagnosis and treatment. With the blend of corrective interventions, SIBO can be effectively managed, improving quality of life, digestive health and overall well-being.

4

What Happens When We 'Kill' Our Gut Feeling?

In Chapter 1, we briefly discussed the vitality of our 'gut feeling' and how it is not just a randomly made-up phrase. In the subsequent chapters, we discussed various factors causing a leaky gut. Now that we have understood what causes a leaky gut, we must understand how a leaky gut manifests mental health issues, a part of which we have already covered in Chapter 1, that is, via the suppression of the production of neurotransmitters. There are a few other facets to it which complete the downward-spiralling cycle, the final few nails in the coffin putting a person inside a dark space, emotionally wounded, disconnected from the world—the last few links connecting the dots, viz. food, gut, brain and mental health.

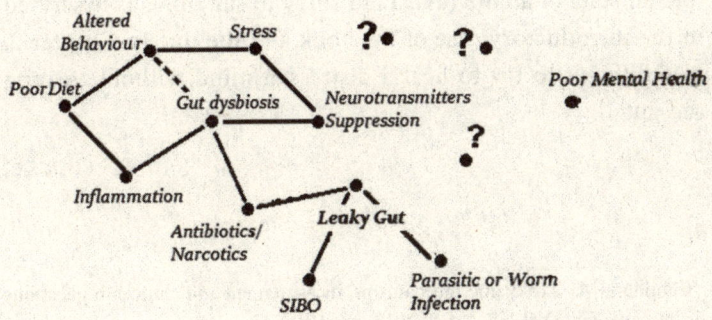

While it is a relatively new concept and some specifics are still being determined, several studies have linked the leaky gut with mood disorders like depression and suicidal ideation, and neurodegenerative diseases such as dementia and Parkinson's across all age groups.[19] Apart from the studies, there are practical examples we bear witness to in our daily lives that show a strong gut-brain-mental-health connection. Having a 'gut-wrenching' experience, feeling 'nauseous' in stressful situations, and feeling 'butterflies' in the stomach are some examples. Another instance is the release of the stomach's juices just by thinking of eating or while food is being served.

The gastrointestinal tract is sensitive to emotion. Anger, anxiety, sadness, elation—all these feelings (and others) can trigger symptoms in the gut. And this connection goes both ways.

Just as a troubled brain can send signals to the gut, a distressed intestine also sends abnormal signals to the brain. Therefore, a person's anxiety, stress or depression can be the result of stomach or intestinal distress. This is especially true in cases where a person experiences mental health issues with no obvious history of financial, professional or personal loss. For such functional abnormality where stress or depression is due to one's own mental state of affairs (and I am sorry to say this), as described in the introductory case of the book and the one in Chapter 2, it is difficult to try to heal a distressed mind without treating the gut.

---

[19] Camilleri, M., 'Leaky gut: mechanisms, measurement and clinical implications in humans', *Gut*, Vol. 68, No. 8, 2019, pp. 1516–26.

The Man Who Could not Catch a Break

If I say this person was a mess when he first came to me, it would be an understatement. He was obese and his overall health was poor. He was diagnosed with fatty liver and diabetes. These metabolic abnormalities culminated in erectile dysfunction. He was suffering from poor sexual health and constantly deteriorating libido for years. It was hard to tell whether his health issues caused problems in his marriage or if it was the other way around. However, there were certainly some indications that both began to happen simultaneously. Consequently, he had no physical or emotional intimacy with his partner, which only worsened his situation.

We knew that his erectile dysfunction was a function of physiological abnormality and emotional imbalances. He was on tadalafil and sildenafil (Viagra) on and off for 10+ years to improve his symptoms. Additionally, he was on other medications to manage his diabetes and fatty liver. Given his marital issues and career crisis, he was also diagnosed with clinical depression and was put on Prozac and sertraline.

We immediately put him on extensive nutritional protocol and botanicals[20] to kick-start his weight loss, improve his fatty liver and treat his diabetes. After six months of careful monitoring and strict compliance, his erectile dysfunction resolved totally. Having gained mental clarity, he became more calm and composed, so much so that his relationship with his wife improved dramatically. Consequently, he stopped taking tadalafil and Viagra as he did not need them anymore. After another few weeks, he was able to stop all his anti-diabetic medications and tapered

---

[20] Botanicals are derived from plants. Specifically, in the health and wellness field, this term refers to plants or parts of plants with medicinal value or health benefits.

down his antidepressants significantly. He remained on botanical supplements for a few more months until he felt motivated and secure, and felt like doing something productive in his life. Thus, it all began with keeping his nutrition in check via diet and botanical supplements.

Leaky Gut to Leaky Brain

Once a pathogen, toxin, microbe (bacteria or fungi), or macromolecule escapes the gut environment through leaky tight junctions, it can travel anywhere in the body upon entering the bloodstream. It's like a wooden plank in the river—it can end up anywhere. This may cause widespread inflammation, including in the brain, causing the breakdown of the blood-brain barrier (BBB) and resulting in a 'leaky brain'. It implies that when the blood-brain barrier is breached, a leaked toxin or pathogen can enter the brain through the blood-brain barrier and attach to vulnerable neurons, generating an immune response from the body and causing further inflammation.

Additionally, inflammation results in cellular and structural changes in the central nervous system and the weakening of synapses—the points through which neurons connect and communicate with each other. When the inflammation persists and becomes chronic, it contributes to neuronal degeneration and promotes a wide array of brain issues causing mental illnesses, and behavioural and neuronal disorders, including, but not limited to, major depression, bipolar disorder, Parkinson's disease, Alzheimer's disease, ADHD, binge eating, and others.

Table: Leaky Gut Causing an Array of Disorders

Neurological Disorders	Eating Disorders
• Parkinson's disease • Alzheimer's disease • Amyotrophic lateral sclerosis (ALS) • Multiple sclerosis	• Anorexia nervosa • Bulimia nervosa • Binge eating disorder
Neurodevelopmental Disorders	**Mental Illness**
• Attention-deficit hyperactivity disorder (ADHD) • Autism spectrum disorder • Cerebral palsy	• Anxiety disorders • Attention-deficit hyperactivity disorder (ADHD) • Depression, bipolar disorder • Obsessive-compulsive disorder (OCD) • Schizophrenia • Suicidal ideation

Let's get into the specifics of it.

When the gut leaks, lipopolysaccharides (LPS) translocate from the organ into blood circulation. LPS, in turn, activates various immune cells, leading to increased secretion of pro-inflammatory cytokines and systemic low-grade inflammation across the physiological systems. Simultaneously, pathogens and toxins released from the leaky gut also evoke an immune response.

The gut houses 70 per cent of our immune system.

So when immune cells feel like there's a threat to the integrity of the gut lining, they sound the alarm by spreading inflammation throughout the body. While a properly controlled immune system acts as a helpful defence mechanism, uncontrolled, chronic and repeated immune responses cause damage and lead to widespread inflammation in the body and brain. During chronic stress or inflammation, tryptophan, a building block for serotonin production, gets deviated to another metabolic pathway[21] instead of producing serotonin. When tryptophan continues down this pathway for a long time, chronic inflammation depletes the body's serotonin and allows toxic substances to be created in the brain. Through this pathway, the leaky gut facilitates the neuroinflammation and neurotransmitter imbalance that we see in the cases of anxiety and depression.

When gut dysbiosis occurs due to poor diet, stress, antibiotics and such others, the leaky gut promotes neurotransmitter imbalance which we often find in relation with abnormal behaviour and cognition in clinical cases of mood disruption, anxiety and depression. Additionally, the interruption of the BBB causes dysfunction of multiple types of neuronal cells, consequently affecting brain function via:

- reducing the number of neurons involved in the production of dopamine,
- disrupting tryptophan metabolism and, in turn, affecting serotonin production, and
- altering the amount of GABA and glutamate, all of which are essential to maintaining mental health.

In a separate mechanism of action, the dysregulation of the gut microbiome that precedes a leaky gut leads to the disruption of the gut's secretion of various types of brain chemicals and proteins, such as brain-derived neurotrophic factor (BDNF). In brief, BDNF is synthesized in both the brain and the gut. It plays an important role in the following:

---

[21]During chronic stress or inflammation, tryptophan is utilized to produce kynurenic acid via the kynurenine pathway.

- Survival and growth of neurons in the gut
- Neurotransmitter modulation in the brain and gut
- Promoting neuronal plasticity in the brain

A disruption or decrease in the levels of BDNF can reduce brain plasticity, and affect its development and even its physical structure. This can lead to issues with memory and learning, and is associated with neurodegeneration and the development of dementia and Alzheimer's.

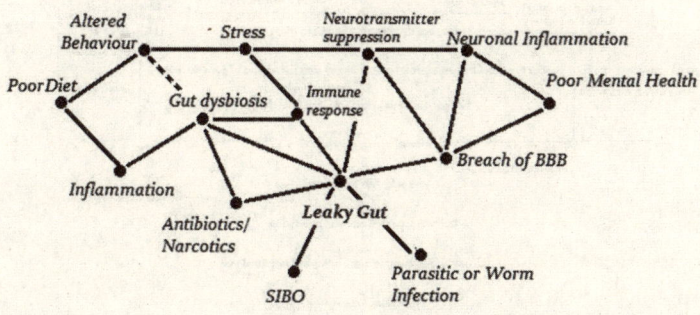

So What Happens When We Kill Our Gut?

All we have been doing is committing a slow suicide, as it has been found, in a literal sense.

A study conducted in 2019 measured the plasma levels of gut permeability markers in patients who had recently attempted suicide, patients with major depression and no history of suicide attempts, and healthy people. Further, the study tried to associate these markers with symptom severity and inflammation. Intestinal permeability was determined in blood plasma by measuring zonulin and intestinal fatty acid-binding protein (I-FABP). The results were astonishing but not surprising. Both zonulin and I-FABP were significantly elevated in patients with a recent suicide attempt.[22] Also, these biomarkers correlated significantly with interleukin-6 (a biomarker of systemic inflammation), clearly indicating that the leaky gut promoted widespread inflammation in the body and contributed to psychiatric issues in a person.

Modelling What We Have Learnt So Far

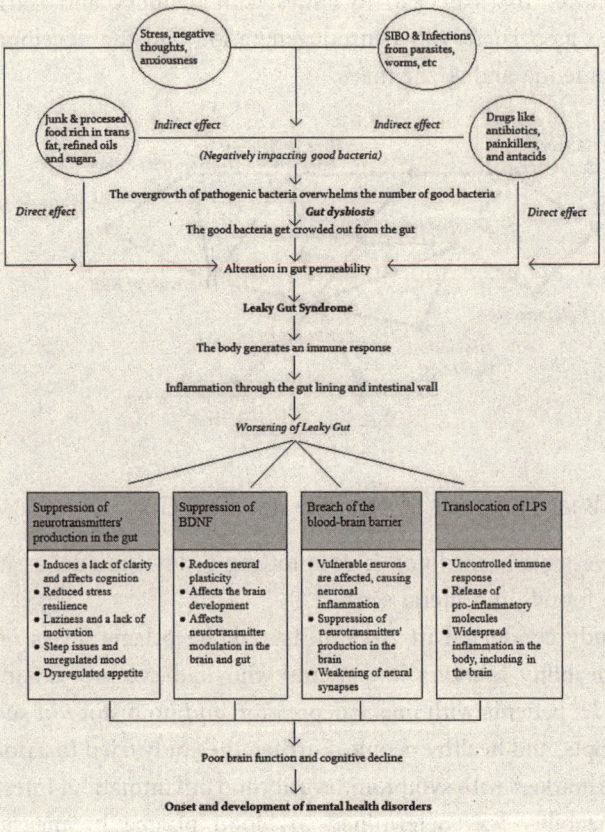

---

[22] Ohlsson, L., et al., 'Leaky gut biomarkers in depression and suicidal behavior', *Acta Psychiatrica Scandinavica*, Vol. 139, No. 2, 2019, pp. 185–93.

All this model represents is the impact of diet, stress, microbial composition, infection and drug use on our gut health and, in turn, our mental health. Consider the neuronal connection (via the vagus nerves) linking the gut and the brain as cables carrying information to and fro through the communication channel of the bloodstream where hormones and inflammation-signalling molecules produced by the gut signal up to the brain. Conversely, the brain uses the hormones it produces to signal down to the gut and affect nerves, smooth muscles and immune cells, modulating their functions.

Gut signals that reach the brain not only generate sensations in the gut (for instance, fullness after having a meal, butterflies in the stomach, a sense of well-being, or nausea and discomfort) but also trigger responses from the brain. When these response signals are sent back to the gut, they generate distinct gut reactions. These responses in the brain and feelings from the gut are stored in vast databases in the brain, which can later be accessed while making decisions—what to eat and drink, whether to fight or run away, chase a goal or leave, with whom to spend time, whether to take up a challenge or quit. What we sense in our gut will ultimately affect how we assess critical information in our relationships, about ourselves and in our careers, be it as a worker, a judge or a leader. An unhealthy gut will send poor signals to the brain, which will generate an unmotivated response (from any aspect, be it immune-system-related or psychosocial). Conversely, a healthy gut will fire up the neurons and generate a proactive response from the brain, getting the job done efficiently and effectively.

The Game of Other Neurotransmitters

In the vast field of what we call the gut-brain axis, there are many neurotransmitters which make it their playground and mount remarkable performances which are pivotal for our mental well-being. Some of these neurotransmitters, as discussed in Chapter 1, are synthesized in the gut, but there are others produced by the central nervous system, inside the brain, or by the glands supporting the nervous system. Among the myriad of these neurotransmitters, four stand out for their profound impact on mental health. These are oxytocin, glutamate, endorphins and histamines. These neurotransmitters, synthesized in the brain and supported by the gut and our diet, are key players in the brain's symphony, influencing everything from happiness to alertness.

Oxytocin: The Bonding Molecule of Love and Trust

Imagine a warm embrace, the joy of holding a newborn, or the comfort of sharing a meaningful conversation with a close friend. These moments of deep connection and trust are made possible, in part, by oxytocin. This molecule is not just a facilitator of social interactions but also a key player in the complex orchestra of emotions that shape our mental well-being.

Often referred to as the 'love hormone' or 'cuddle hormone', oxytocin is a remarkable substance that plays a crucial role in human connection, trust and emotional bonding. It's a hormone and neurotransmitter that has fascinated scientists and laypeople alike for its profound impact on social behaviours, emotional regulation and mental health. It is produced in the hypothalamus, a region of the brain responsible for many vital functions, including the regulation of emotions, appetite and the body's stress response. From the hypothalamus, oxytocin is released into the bloodstream by the pituitary gland, or it acts directly within the brain as a neurotransmitter, facilitating communication between neurons.

Impact on Mental Health

Oxytocin is best known for its role in childbirth and lactation. During labour, oxytocin levels surge, helping to induce contractions and facilitate the delivery of the baby. After birth, oxytocin stimulates milk production, fostering the crucial bond between mother and child. Beyond these well-known roles, oxytocin's influence extends to various aspects of our social behaviour and emotional well-being:

- **Bonding and Attachment:** Oxytocin is often called the 'bonding hormone' because of its ability to promote feelings of closeness and connection. It is essential for the formation of social bonds, whether between parents and children, romantic partners, or even friends.
- **Trust and Empathy:** Oxytocin enhances feelings of trust and empathy, making it easier for individuals to connect with others on an emotional level. This hormone is often released during positive social interactions, reinforcing feelings of trust and cooperation.
- **Stress Reduction:** Oxytocin has a calming effect on the brain, helping to reduce anxiety and stress. It counters the effects of cortisol, the stress hormone, and promotes a sense of relaxation and security.
- **Emotional Regulation:** Oxytocin helps regulate emotions by modulating activity in the brain's limbic system, the area responsible for emotional responses. This can lead to improved mood, reduced fear, and a greater ability to cope with challenging situations.

Oxytocin's role in mental health is profound. High levels of oxytocin are associated with positive emotional states, such as happiness, calmness and trust. It has been found to be particularly important in managing stress and anxiety. For instance, studies have shown that oxytocin can help reduce social anxiety, enhance feelings of safety, and improve social interactions.

Furthermore, oxytocin has therapeutic potential for conditions such as depression, post-traumatic stress disorder (PTSD) and autism spectrum disorders, where social functioning and emotional regulation are often impaired. By enhancing social bonding and reducing stress, oxytocin can contribute to better mental health and overall well-being.

While oxytocin is primarily released in response to physical touch, positive social interactions and certain hormonal signals, certain foods and lifestyle choices can support the overall environment in which oxytocin production occurs. The foods include dark chocolate, avocados, omega-3-rich foods like desi ghee, seeds (chia seeds and flaxseeds), and salmon, and foods rich in vitamin C like broccoli. We will get into the details of dietary sources in the Part 2 of the book as well.

Glutamate: A Neurotransmitter of Neurotransmitters

Glutamate is an amino acid that is made by the glial cells in your brain and serves as the most abundant excitatory neurotransmitter[23] found in the body. Most importantly, it is responsible for the synthesis of GABA and in the modulation of synaptic plasticity[24] and neurotransmission.

---

[23] Excitatory neurotransmitters 'excite' the neuron and cause it to 'fire off the message', meaning the message continues to be passed along to the next cell.

[24] 'Synaptic or neural plasticity' refers to the capacity of the nervous system to modify itself, functionally and structurally, in response to experience and injury. It serves as an essential phenomenon for learning and developing memory.

> *Think of glutamate as a neurotransmitters' neurotransmitter—it helps transmit a message that primarily excites other neurons to release their neurotransmitters.*

Multiple studies have found abnormalities in the metabolic pathways synthesizing or using glutamate in patients with depression. There is now emerging evidence linking alterations in glutamate levels and dysregulation of glutamate signalling with the onset and progression of disorders like depression, autism, epilepsy and schizophrenia.[25]

Impact on Mental Health

By mediating the strengthening and reorganization of neural connections, glutamate has been found to play a key role in:

- Enhancing cognition and mental clarity, and suppressing cognitive or mental fatigue
- Regulating mood and modulating stress resilience
- Improving learning and memory

Glutamate, apart from being synthesized in our body, is also derived from dietary sources such as cheese, meat and additives like monosodium glutamate.

Endorphins: The Brain's Natural Painkillers

Endorphins are a group of neurotransmitters produced by the central nervous system and the pituitary gland. The name 'endorphin' comes from 'endogenous morphine', which highlights their primary function—acting as the body's natural painkillers.

---

[25] Onaolapo, A.Y., and O.J. Onaolapo, 'Glutamate and depression: Reflecting a deepening knowledge of the gut and brain effects of a ubiquitous molecule', *World Journal of Psychiatry*, Vol. 11, No. 7, 2021, pp. 297–315.

They are part of the brain's reward system, helping to reduce pain and induce feelings of pleasure or euphoria.

Impact on Mental Health

Endorphins are most famously known for their role in the 'runner's high'—a feeling of euphoria experienced after intense physical activity. However, their influence extends far beyond just physical exercise. When endorphins are released, they interact with receptors in the brain to reduce the perception of pain, much like opioid drugs but without the harmful side effects. This interaction not only helps in pain management but also promotes a sense of well-being and happiness. Endorphins also play a crucial role in:

- Reducing stress, anxiety and depression
- Modulating appetite
- The release of sex hormones
- Enhancing immune response

A deficiency in endorphins can lead to chronic pain, depression and a lack of enjoyment in life, underscoring their importance in maintaining mental and emotional balance.

Histamines: The Body's Alertness Agents

Histamines are another group of neurotransmitters but they are more commonly known for their role in allergic reactions. Produced by cells called mast cells, histamines are released in response to allergens, leading to symptoms like itching, sneezing and swelling. However, their role in the body is far more complex and extends into the realm of neurotransmission.

Impact on Mental Health

Histamines help keep the brain alert and awake, contributing to a state of readiness and focus. This makes them crucial for maintaining attention and preventing drowsiness. They play a crucial role in:

- Regulating the sleep-wake cycle
- Modulating appetite
- Maintaining cognitive functions such as learning and memory
- Regulating mood

An imbalance in histamine levels can contribute to conditions such as anxiety, depression and even schizophrenia. For example, low levels of histamine are associated with excessive sleepiness and reduced cognitive function, while high levels can contribute to anxiety and hyperactivity.

Understanding the Biopsychosocial Model

So far, we have been blaming poor diet and a stressful lifestyle for the leaky gut and the mental health issues it induces. But we cannot overlook the complex interplay of biological, psychological and other social factors that can also exacerbate symptoms of psychiatric disorders.

In brief, the biopsychosocial model of mental health emphasizes the interaction between biological, psychological and social factors in shaping mental health and illness. According to this model, mental health issues can arise from different permutations and combinations of biological vulnerabilities, psychological processes and environmental stressors, including lifestyle factors. While this book addresses biological vulnerabilities and lifestyle factors, we have not discussed in detail the depression caused by past trauma, adverse childhood experiences, personality traits, loss of loved ones or financial loss, though such psychological factors also interact with lifestyle choices and environmental stressors (as in the case discussed in this chapter), contributing to the complexity of mental health conditions.

Generally, psychiatrists use medications as a first line of treatment and psychologists focus on counselling alone. However, these forms of treatment do not address environmental stressors, including poor diet, a sedentary lifestyle and stressful daily activities, which I believe are the stimulus for the development of underlying depressive symptoms. So why is it that patients do not respond well to treatment and have to be put on antidepressants for a lifetime? Why could a therapeutic method not induce behavioural changes in patients seeking help to get well?

Could a Leaky Gut Be the Reason for Treatment-Resistant Depression?

Just like you cannot outrun a bad diet, you cannot out-medicate depression, at least not every time. And sometimes, you don't even require medication to begin with, *which is what we will deal with in Part 2 of the book*. SSRI medications such as Zoloft and Lexapro can help reduce symptoms of depression caused by low serotonin levels, which could have been the result of widespread inflammation and the activation of the kynurenine pathway due to a leaky gut. When that's the case, medications ultimately do not address the full cascade of events seen with a leaky gut. Consequently, patients might feel better for a short while but their symptoms never resolve completely. If your depression symptoms have been lingering for a while even after starting the treatment, you might want to see a provider or therapist who considers the role of the gut-brain axis in mental health and looks beyond chemical imbalances in the brain, as the root cause of your health issues might not be in your brain but somewhere else.

Keep in Mind: The Dynamic Human-Microbe Cycle

All in all, poor diet and stress go hand in hand to cause gut dysbiosis, which then triggers an immune response and inflammation in a neverending loop. Chronic use of antibiotics or narcotics, SIBO, or recurring infections can also cause gut dysbiosis, ultimately leading to the leaky gut phenomenon. Toxins and pathogens released from a leaky gut can end up anywhere in the body including the brain. They breach the blood-brain barrier, suppress neuronal activity and cause neuronal inflammation. This generates an immune response from the body and causes further inflammation.

Stress and depression alter the gut microbiota via immune, neuronal/neurotransmitters and hormonal signalling. On the other hand, our food choices and dietary habits help to determine which bacteria flourish—probiotics or pathogens. Stress and depression can provoke dysregulated eating, and conversely, diet modulates stress reactivity and mood. It implies that diet and stress can engage with each other, governing the gut environment together. Additionally, the gut microbes either directly secrete or help release metabolites, toxins and neurohormones, which either promote inflammation or enhance our well-being. Depending on our diet, dominant bacterial species may promote their own interests over those of humans by releasing molecules that mimic appetite hormones, thereby fuelling food cravings. Through this diet-mediated path, the gut microbiome impacts our overall mood, behaviour, and responses to stress. Ultimately, the individual's stressors, mood and diet, coupled with their gut bacteria, can alter their immune function and health.

PART 2

Healing from Within: Building a Healthier Relationship with Food

Now that we have established the roles of gut dysbiosis and leaky gut in disturbing mental health, an obvious question arises, '*What can we do to prevent leaky gut and promote mental health?*' The foremost answer is very simple: a good-quality, balanced and nutritious diet. And we will elaborate on that throughout Part 2 of this book.

Ayurvedic dietary principles have profoundly influenced cultural attitudes towards food and wellness in India and beyond. Traditional Indian cuisine reflects the principles of Ayurveda, with an emphasis on whole grains, legumes, vegetables and spices prepared in ways that enhance digestion and flavour. Moreover, Ayurvedic rituals such as mindful eating, cooking with intention, and fasting are deeply ingrained in Indian cultural practices, fostering a holistic approach to nourishment and self-care.

Following the principles of Ayurveda and modern scientific research, I've realized that they are directing us toward similar foods— whole grains, naturally occurring good fats, vegetables, herbs and spices, and nuts and seeds.

Hi there,

It's me, Social Media, again! I see you've met many interesting characters by now through your journey into this book—such as serotonin, dopamine, GABA, BDNF, HNF-4 alpha, glutamate, and others. You're way better informed than when we last met. You've got everything you need to know about the onset and progression of mental health issues. Now you will get everything you need to know about fixing it.

By the looks of it, the solution would be simple yet complex, easy but something that requires stringency, but most importantly, is doable. The best part is that you have now '*cut the noise*'

> facilitated by me, and will continue to do so while you find solutions to the mental health issues and challenges discussed in Part 1.
>
> Despite the growing interest in the therapeutic impact of food on the nervous system and mental health, the details available on food sources for neurotransmitters are inadequate, which is where this book intends to fill a few gaps. Part 2 offers practical strategies and lifestyle changes to optimize gut health and potentially alleviate mental health symptoms. You will become aware of dietary interventions, including the intake of probiotics, prebiotics and micronutrient-rich food contributing to the healing of the gut and boosting the intake, production, availability and functions of neurotransmitters, thus improving mental health.
>
> By now, you've understood how poor diet, stress and uncontrolled use of antibiotics or narcotics manifest in mental health issues by affecting the gut-brain connection. Moving further, you will come to know how you can fix these issues 'mindfully' by incorporating healthy and nutritious food in your diet, and changing the way you eat in a manner that reignites your relationship with food and fosters a deeper connection with the phenomenon of eating. By the end of the book, you will no longer eat just to fill your tummy, but extract so many positive things from it that would also impact the state of your mind.

Reiterating the Importance of Gut Health

At birth, every gut is sterile. Over time, our guts develop a diverse and distinct brew of microbial species, including bacteria, fungi and protozoa. The gut microenvironment is determined partly by genetics and partly by the kind of microbes living in and around us. The 100 trillion microbes inside the gut are critical to our health as they regulate digestion, metabolism, immunity, inflammation, mental health and overall well-being. However, a gut is considered healthy only when it has an enriched diversity of beneficial bacteria which outnumber harmful bacteria.

Good microbes extract, assimilate and synthesize vitamins and other nutrients from the food we eat. They produce metabolites that enable them to programme the body's immune system while building and maintaining the gut wall which protects the body from outside invaders. By their very presence, probiotics (good bacteria) in the gut block harmful microbes from setting up camp and produce anti-microbial chemicals that defend the host against pathogens.

A healthy gut produces hundreds of neurochemicals which the brain utilizes to regulate primary physiological and mental processes such as learning, memory and mood. As discussed earlier, gut bacteria manufacture about 95 per cent of the body's serotonin supply, which influences mood and GI activity. Keep in mind the gut's multifaceted ability to communicate with the brain and set up the body's immunity to defend against threats from the outside world. When you consider this, it is unimaginable to think that the gut does not play a significant role in regulating the states of the mind and mental health.

So how do we ensure gut health? Our gut needs probiotics… and…probiotics need prebiotics.

Probiotics refer to a set of microbes acting beneficially, particularly for their host. In humans, these good bacteria reside in the gut (small and large intestines). On the other hand, prebiotics are a group of nutrients upon which our gut microbiome acts, degrading them into products with a range of benefits—from digestion to developing better immunity. For instance, inulin, fructooligosaccharides (FOS), and galacto-oligosaccharides (GOS) are a few compounds that serve as prebiotics. Their degradation via fermentation by gut microbiota yields short-chain fatty acids (SCFAs) including lactic acid, butyric acid and propionic acid.

Highlighting the science, the International Scientific Association of Probiotics and Prebiotics (ISAPP) defined 'dietary prebiotics' as '**a selectively fermented ingredient that results in specific changes in the composition and/or activity of the gastrointestinal microbiota, thus conferring benefit(s) upon host health**'.[26] Prebiotics modulate the composition and function of probiotic bacteria by serving as energy sources for them, thus rejuvenating gut microbiota. Certain kinds of foods have a blend of prebiotics for the bacteria living in our gut.

First and foremost, we need to set our meals right and prioritize eating wholesome, freshly cooked and protein-rich food over junk and processed food. And this is what we will keep our focus on throughout the book. In Part 1, we discussed major factors causing poor gut health, including food, stress, chronic use of antibiotics or narcotics, SIBO and parasitic infections. A good-quality, nutritious diet can negate the ill-effects of all the other factors. Healthy food choices and dietary habits can:

- help modulate stress resilience and increase our ability to cope with stressful situations in a much better way
- boost our immunity to fight infections efficiently and control inflammatory responses, preventing gut leakage
- suppress the ill-effects of antibiotics by boosting the growth of probiotics and strengthening the integrity of the gut lining

---

[26]Davani-Davari, D., et al., 'Prebiotics: Definition, Types, Sources, Mechanisms, and Clinical Applications', *Foods*, Vol. 8, No. 3, 2019, p. 92.

- suppress the ill-effects of narcotics by improving gut motility and controlling systemic inflammation via boosting the immune function
- prevent SIBO by improving gut motility and modulating stress responses

Stress, antibiotics or narcotics, SIBO and gut infections can all foster a leaky gut via different mechanisms, i.e. by altering immune function, causing dysbiosis, or directly affecting intestinal permeability. Conversely, a healthy diet boosts immune responses, controls inflammation and strengthens the gut lining. It implies that nutritious food can suppress, negate and reverse the detrimental physiological effects caused by stress, drugs, SIBO or infections.

In the upcoming chapters, we will look into:

- foods comprising a rich blend of prebiotic compounds
- foods that can serve as an affluent source of probiotics to enhance gut health
- the nutrient profile that can serve as a base for improving gut health and brain function, thus boosting our states of mind

Eating bad-quality, non-nutritious food is one part of the problem. Eating mindlessly and overeating is another facet of it. So eating right will solve 80 per cent of the problem. To completely ensure our gut health, resolve our mental health issues, and prevent them from recurring, we also need to understand how to eat right. The latter half of Part 2 will discuss how to eat using our minds to make the food positively affect mind states.

It's high time we awakened our body's wisdom to listen to the signal it is trying to send. Only then can we honour our hunger and make peace with the food that nature is offering, enabling us to suppress cravings and discover the satisfaction factor of food.

By engaging our senses, slowing down, and listening to our bodies, we can break free from the cycle of mindless overeating, and embrace a more balanced and fulfilling approach to nourishment. An awareness of the impact of both processed and healthy (nutritious) foods on our brain chemistry empowers us to make informed choices that prioritize our well-being over fleeting pleasure, which is what we attempt to create in Part 2 of the book.

5

Heal Your Gut, Heal Your Mind: A Plate Full of Prebiotics and Probiotics

Imagine waking up each morning feeling energized and ready to take on the day. Picture yourself free from the fog of fatigue and the grip of mood swings that often disrupt your daily life. You are so clear-headed that you know exactly what you want to achieve in a day or get things done by people at work. You know the risks you are taking and if things go wrong, you are already prepared for it. Basically, you have it all planned out! How happy or relaxed would you be if that were the state of your mind all the time, or say, at least most of the time? What if the key to unlocking this vibrant state of health lies in your kitchen—something as simple as the food on your plate?

The intricate relationship between the gut and the brain—the gut-brain axis—highlights how the state of our digestive system can affect our mood, cognition and mental clarity. Healing your gut is not just about dietary changes; it's about adopting a holistic approach to nurturing your digestive system and, in turn, fostering a healthier mind. Remember the line on promoting and rejuvenating gut health: *Our gut needs Probiotics…and…Probiotics need Prebiotics*. There are two parts to the answer—prebiotics and probiotics.

Probiotics in the gut thrive on prebiotics. Conversely, pathogens thrive on simple sugars.

We must either feed our gut prebiotics to promote the growth of probiotics or directly take in adequate amounts of probiotic microbes. The ingestion of vibrant probiotics causes vital improvements in balancing intestinal permeability and barrier function, thus preventing or treating the leaky gut syndrome. For instance, fermented food products are home to probiotic bacteria. On the other hand, natural, wholesome foods containing a blend of non-digestable fermentable compounds (like inulin, FOS and GOS) serve as prebiotic food, promoting the survival of good bacteria and suppressing pathogenic growth.

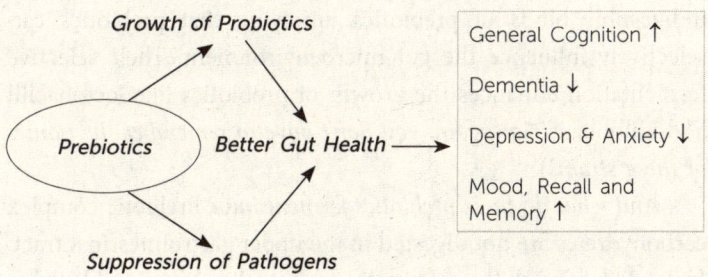

Subsequently, a good-quality diet will remove pathogenic bacteria and maintain gut stability. And let me tell you, almost all the ingredients you need to design your daily plate with healthy nutritious food—complete with prebiotics and probiotics—are present in your kitchen or readily available in the market closest to your home. So let's start plating!

Prebiotics for Gut Health

The gut environment is a complex ecosystem where trillions of microorganisms coexist and play a vital role in human health.

The fermentation of complex carbohydrates by gut bacteria is a critical process in maintaining the stability of this ecosystem and the integrity of the gut lining. Among the best-researched prebiotics are inulin, fructooligosaccharides (FOS) and galacto-oligosaccharides (GOS). Inulin, FOS and GOS can greatly modify the composition and function of gut microbiota. All these prebiotics are resistant to upper gastrointestinal (GI) digestion.

Biochemically, prebiotics are nothing but complex carbohydrates, also called dietary fibres. These terms are often used interchangeably for the same compounds: inulin, FOS and GOS.

Beneficial gut microbiota ferment these non-digestible prebiotics in the colon and obtain their survival energy from degrading indigestible binds of prebiotics, implying that prebiotics can selectively influence the gut microenvironment. Their selective fermentation enhances the growth of probiotics like lactobacilli and bifidobacteria (*again, you don't have to remember the names of these strains*).

And what do these prebiotics ferment into? Prebiotic complex carbohydrates are not digested in the upper gastrointestinal tract. Instead, they reach the colon intact, where they become substrates for fermentation by good gut bacteria. This process of anaerobic fermentation[27] primarily involves the breakdown of fibres like inulin, GOS, FOS, resistant starches, pectins and other non-digestible carbohydrates. These dietary fibres are fermented into smaller compounds like short-chain fatty acids (SCFAs) including lactic acid, butyric acid and propionic acid. These products can have multiple effects on the body—from enhancing gut health

---

[27] A process where microorganisms, primarily in the gut, break down complex carbohydrates without the presence of oxygen, producing energy and metabolites.

and boosting the immune system to enhancing brain function. This is because SCFAs can diffuse in our blood circulation and affect not only the gut but also distant organs.

A Short Note on SCFAs

One of the most critical outcomes of carbohydrate fermentation is the production of SCFAs including acetate, propionate and butyrate. These SCFAs serve several vital functions:

- **Energy Source for Colonocytes:** Butyrate, in particular, is a primary energy source for the cells lining the colon (colonocytes). By providing energy, butyrate helps maintain the health and function of the gut lining, promoting a strong barrier against pathogens and toxins.
- **Regulation of pH:** SCFAs support gut health by lowering the pH of the gut, inhibiting the growth of pathogenic bacteria and fostering a more favourable habitat for beneficial microbes, thereby maintaining microbial balance.
- **Anti-Inflammatory Properties:** SCFAs exhibit anti-inflammatory properties, reducing the risk of inflammatory bowel diseases and other gut-related disorders.

By reducing systemic inflammation, SCFAs help mitigate neuroinflammation, a factor linked to mental health disorders such as depression and anxiety. SCFAs, particularly acetate, can cross the blood-brain barrier and influence the synthesis of neurotransmitters like serotonin and dopamine, which are crucial for mood regulation and mental health. They also affect the hypothalamic-pituitary-adrenal (HPA) axis. Now, consider the HPA axis as the body's stress response system. This system, via a chain of reactions, releases a key stress hormone called cortisol in response to a threat or stress. Cortisol helps the body manage stress by increasing energy availability, suppressing non-essential functions, and modulating the immune response. Once the stressor is dealt with, cortisol levels typically drop and the HPA axis returns to its baseline state.

However, chronic stress can disrupt this balance. The persistent activation of the HPA axis leads to consistently high levels of cortisol, which can result in several health issues including anxiety, depression, immune system suppression and metabolic disorders. Over time, the HPA axis can become dysregulated, leading to either hyperactivation (excessive cortisol production) or hypoactivation (insufficient cortisol production), both of which can exacerbate stress-related conditions. Countering this detrimental condition, SCFAs play a role in maintaining the balance of the HPA axis. They support the integrity of the gut barrier and influence the gut-brain axis, which in turn helps modulate the release of cortisol and the body's response to stress, and potentially reduces symptoms of stress-related mental health conditions.

Availability of Prebiotics

The human diet is the chief source of prebiotics, providing energy for the growth of probiotics. Many wholesome foods act as natural sources of prebiotics.

So where can we get prebiotics naturally?

Foods like asparagus, garlic, chicory, onion, Jerusalem artichoke, wheat, honey, banana, barley, tomato, rye, soybean, human and cow's milk, peas, beans, and such others serve as natural sources of prebiotics. Most of these foods contain prebiotics in low concentration, which is why we, as nutritionists, have to depend on pharmaceutical-grade prebiotic supplements to kickstart a treatment. However, there are a few selective foods that offer prebiotics in relatively high amounts and we will discuss them now.

Garlic

- **Benefits for Gut Health**: It contains inulin, a type of fibre that promotes the growth of beneficial gut bacteria.
- **Benefits for Mental Health**: Rich in antioxidants that can help reduce inflammation and oxidative stress, potentially improving mood and cognitive function.

Onions

- **Benefits for Gut Health**: High in fructooligosaccharides (FOS) which feed the good bacteria in the gut.
- **Benefits for Mental Health**: Contains quercetin, an antioxidant that may help reduce symptoms of anxiety and depression.

Asparagus

- **Benefits for Gut Health**: Packed with inulin, which enhances gut flora.
- **Benefits for Mental Health**: High in folate which is essential for brain function and has been linked to a reduced risk of depression.

Bananas

- **Benefits for Gut Health**: Contains resistant starch and pectin, both of which act as prebiotics.
- **Benefits for Mental Health**: Is a good source of

vitamin B6, which helps synthesize neurotransmitters like serotonin, oxytocin and dopamine which are crucial for mood regulation.

Ginger

- **Benefits for Gut Health**: Its biological active compound 6-gingerol exhibits prebiotic properties by promoting the growth of specific beneficial strains of bacteria such as *Lactobacillus* in the gut, thus promoting gut health. It also enhances gastric motility and can help in the efficient movement of food through the digestive tract, reducing symptoms of bloating and discomfort.
- **Benefits for Mental Health**: Is a good source of vitamin B6, which helps synthesize neurotransmitters like serotonin and dopamine, crucial for mood regulation. It also helps boost the production of endorphins which can help reduce stress.

Leeks

- **Benefits for Gut Health**: High in inulin; it supports a healthy gut microbiome.
- **Benefits for Mental Health**: Contains kaempferol, a flavonoid with potential anti-inflammatory and neuroprotective effects.

Jerusalem Artichokes

- **Benefits for Gut Health**: Also known as sunchokes, they are rich in inulin, fostering good gut bacteria.
- **Benefits for Mental Health**: High in potassium and iron which are important for brain function and energy levels.

Chicory Root

- **Benefits for Gut Health**: One of the richest sources of inulin, promoting beneficial gut bacteria.
- **Benefits for Mental Health**: Helps improve digestion and the absorption of nutrients essential for brain health.

Dandelion Greens (*Sinhaparni*)

Dandelions are a part of the sunflower family.

- **Benefits for Gut Health**: Contains high levels of fibre and inulin.
- **Benefits for Mental Health**: Rich in antioxidants and vitamins A and C, which support overall brain health and reduce oxidative stress.

Apples

- **Benefits for Gut Health**: High in pectin, which increases butyrate, a short-chain fatty acid that feeds beneficial gut bacteria.
- **Benefits for Mental Health**: Is a good source of quercetin and vitamin C, both of which have neuroprotective properties.

Barley

- **Benefits for Gut Health**: Contains beta-glucan, a prebiotic fibre that promotes healthy gut bacteria.
- **Benefits for Mental Health**: High in selenium, which helps protect against oxidative damage and supports cognitive function.

Incorporating these prebiotic-rich foods into your diet can support a healthy gut microbiome and enhance your mental health through improved nutrient absorption, reduced inflammation and better neurotransmitter production.

Unmasking Mental Health: A Patient's Journey beyond Medication

'Emma'[28], a 32-year-old woman, was struggling with anxiety and depression for several years when she came to me. Despite being on medication and undergoing therapy, Emma felt that her mental health issues were not fully resolved. She approached me for nutritional guidance to complement her existing treatment.

The journey of guiding patients towards a healthier lifestyle can often be filled with moments of surprise and revelation. Whenever I recommend patients a diet that incorporates prebiotics and foods rich in micronutrients, people look at me bemused. The room often fills up with astonishment and curiosity. '*I already eat a lot of vegetables and lentils,*' one patient might say, eyes wide with surprise. Another might chime in, '*I use garlic and onions all the time. Why haven't I seen any improvements?*' It's a common reaction. Emma's reaction was the same. She could not fathom how these foods could improve her mental health when none of the medications worked, and especially when she had been eating them since childhood. So I asked her the following:

- '*How many times a day you eat junk food or go to fancy restaurants for a meal with your family or friends?*' Her answer actually astonished me, '*every other day.*'
- '*The cooking oil you use at home?*' Her reply was '*sunflower or soybean refined oil.*'
- '*The number of times you reheat your cooked lentils or vegetables?*' She replied, '*2–3 times.*'

---

[28]Name changed for privacy.

When I get these types of answers, I know for a fact that people at home are not getting much nutrition despite eating healthy food. And whatever nutrition they get is compromised by the inclusion of junk food or foods that promote the production of inflammatory molecules. And yes, I am talking about the refined oils we use plenty of times and in decent amounts every day. Plant-based refined oils contain trans fats and omega-6 fatty acids which are linked to increased inflammation, cardiovascular diseases and other chronic conditions.

Additionally, overcooking vegetables can lead to a significant loss of water-soluble vitamins (like vitamin C and B vitamins) and heat-sensitive nutrients. High-temperature cooking methods such as frying can lead to the formation of acrylamides and other harmful compounds that only deteriorate gut health by compromising the integrity of gut lining and supporting pathogen growth. Furthermore, reheating food multiple times further degrades the food quality and strips the food of whatever nutrient content is left.

Initial Assessment

During my initial consultation with Emma, I conducted a comprehensive assessment, which included:

- **Dietary Habits**: Her diet was relatively low in fibre and high in processed foods, which negatively impacted her gut health.
- **Symptoms**: She reported frequent gastrointestinal issues, including bloating, constipation and discomfort, alongside symptoms of anxiety and depression.
- **Lifestyle**: Despite being outgoing, Emma otherwise led a sedentary lifestyle working from home, with irregular sleep patterns adding to her overall stress levels.

Based on my assessment, I devised a nutrition plan focused on incorporating prebiotic-rich foods and supplements to support gut health with the aim of positively influencing her mental health through the gut-brain axis.

1. Dietary Changes

- **Garlic and Onion**: I recommended adding raw or lightly cooked garlic and onions to her meals. These foods are rich in inulin and FOS which are effective prebiotics.
- **Ginger**: Emma started incorporating fresh ginger into her diet, adding it to smoothies, teas and various dishes. Ginger not only has prebiotic properties but also offers anti-inflammatory benefits.
- **Chicory Root**: I suggested she replace her morning coffee with a chicory root beverage which is high in inulin and can support gut health.
- **Fermented Foods**: To further enhance the diversity of her gut microbiota, I encouraged the inclusion of fermented foods like yogurt, kefir, sauerkraut and kimchi.
- **Whole Foods**: I emphasized the importance of a diet rich in whole foods, including plenty of vegetables, fruits, whole grains and legumes.

2. Prebiotic Supplements

- I prescribed a high-quality prebiotic supplement containing inulin, FOS and GOS to ensure she received adequate amounts of these beneficial fibres.

3. Lifestyle Modifications

- **Physical Activity**: I advised Emma to engage in regular physical activity such as daily walks or yoga to help

manage stress and improve gut motility.
- **Sleep Hygiene**: We discussed strategies for improving her sleep patterns, such as establishing a regular bedtime routine and reducing screen time before bed.

Progress and Outcome

1. Short-Term Improvements

- Within a few weeks, Emma reported reduced gastrointestinal discomfort. The bloating and constipation she previously experienced began to diminish.
- She also noticed slight improvements in her mood and energy levels, which motivated her to adhere to the nutritional plan.

2. Long-Term Benefits

- After three months, Emma experienced significant improvements in her anxiety and depression symptoms. Her mood was more stable and she had fewer episodes of intense anxiety.
- The combination of dietary changes and prebiotic supplements led to a more balanced gut microbiota, which was confirmed by a follow-up gut microbiome test.
- Emma's sleep quality improved, further contributing to her overall mental well-being.

3. Sustained Lifestyle Changes

- Emma continued to incorporate prebiotic-rich foods into her diet and maintained the lifestyle modifications. She reported feeling more in control of her mental health and overall wellness.

This case highlights the profound impact of dietary interventions, specifically the inclusion of prebiotic-rich foods and supplements, on mental health. By improving gut health through the use of garlic, ginger, onion, chicory root and prebiotic supplements, we were able to support Emma's journey towards better mental health. People think of these foods as ordinary, but what they don't realize is their prolific micronutrient profile. And when these ordinary foods are eaten without any adulteration from refined oils and junk food, they can create magic to boost good health (something which I have discussed in my previous book Heal with Foods: Magical Ingredients That Will Change Your Life). *It is worth noting that prebiotic-rich foods also contain an abundance of micronutrients and amino acids that are essential for boosting mental health (which we will discuss in the next chapter). Additionally, many of these foods are used in the preparation of probiotics-rich food. Hence, you will find references to the above-listed foods in the next segment as well as the next chapter.*

Fermented Products as the Source of Probiotics

Technically speaking, fermentation is an anaerobic process where microbes like bacteria and yeast feed upon, metabolize and break down carbohydrates (sugar and starch), proteins and fats into simpler substances (byproducts), such as alcohol-based products and organic acids (for example, lactic acid and acetic acid). These alcohol-based products do not necessarily mean liquor. Fermented foods and beverages are products made via fermentation with the help of controlled microbial growth. The phrase '**controlled microbial growth**' is of significance as this ensures quality and prevents spoilage while offering a large enough concentration of probiotic bacteria or yeast in the food. This process not only preserves the food but also enhances its nutritional profile and flavour.

Fermented products like yogurt, kefir, kimchi, sauerkraut and kombucha have been cherished for centuries across various cultures for their unique flavours and health benefits. These foods are not only delicious but also serve as natural probiotics, providing a wealth of benefits for gut health and overall well-being.

But how exactly do fermented products function as probiotics? Let's delve into the science behind these culinary staples and uncover their transformative potential for our health.

The Science behind Fermented Foods

Fermented foods and beverages are rich in beneficial bacteria and yeasts. When ingested, they interact positively with the gut microbiota and form symbiotic relationships. Common probiotic strains found in these foods include:

- *Lactobacillus*: Often found in yogurt and kefir
- *Bifidobacterium*: Common in dairy products
- *Saccharomyces*: A type of beneficial yeast found in fermented beverages like kombucha

Common examples of fermented products include:

- **Yogurt:** Made by fermenting milk with lactic acid bacteria, primarily Lactobacillus bulgaricus and *Streptococcus thermophilus*
- **Kimchi:** A traditional Korean dish of fermented vegetables, typically including cabbage and radishes, seasoned with chili pepper, garlic, ginger and other spices
- **Sauerkraut:** Fermented cabbage that undergoes lactic acid fermentation, resulting in a tangy, crunchy side dish
- **Kombucha:** A fermented tea beverage made using a ***symbiotic culture of bacteria and yeast (SCOBY)***

You don't have to remember the names of probiotic strains, but you can understand the science behind how they enhance gut health.

1. Colonization of the Gut

- Probiotics from fermented foods can temporarily colonize the gut, contributing to the overall microbial population. While they might not permanently alter the gut microbiota, they interact with the resident microbiota to enhance their function.

2. Competitive Exclusion

- Probiotics compete with pathogenic bacteria for nutrients and adhesion sites on the gut lining. This competition helps prevent the overgrowth of harmful bacteria, thus maintaining a balanced gut microbiota.

3. Production of Antimicrobial Substances

- Probiotics produce substances like bacteriocins, hydrogen peroxide and organic acids (for example, lactic acid) that inhibit the growth of pathogenic bacteria. These antimicrobial compounds help to control harmful microorganisms in the gut.

4. Modulation of the Immune System

- Probiotics interact with the gut-associated lymphoid tissue (GALT) to modulate immune responses. They can enhance the production of anti-inflammatory cytokines and reduce the production of pro-inflammatory cytokines, contributing to immune regulation and reducing the risk of chronic inflammation.

5. Enhancement of the Gut Barrier Function

- Probiotics strengthen the gut barrier by increasing the production of mucus and enhancing tight junctions between epithelial cells. This barrier prevents pathogens and toxins from entering the bloodstream, reducing the risk of systemic infections and inflammation.

6. Metabolic Functions

- Probiotics help in the digestion of food and absorption of nutrients. They produce SCFAs such as butyrate, acetate and propionate during the fermentation of dietary fibres. SCFAs serve as an energy source for colonocytes and exhibit anti-inflammatory effects, promoting gut health. SCFAs, especially propionate, help regulate blood sugar levels by influencing insulin sensitivity and reducing glucose production in the liver. This can aid in preventing and managing conditions like type 2 diabetes.
- Probiotics also play a role in regulating lipid metabolism by boosting the production of digestive enzymes, and promoting the absorption and utilization of molecules that help reduce triglycerides[29] production in the liver, which can contribute to cardiovascular health.

Mental Health Benefits of Fermented Foods

Resident microbial species as well as final biomolecular products like organic acids and alcohols help preserve fermented foods for a long duration, and endow them with their unique aroma,

---

[29] Triglycerides are a type of fat (lipid) found in your blood. High triglycerides contribute to hardening of the arteries or thickening of the artery walls, known as arteriosclerosis.

desirable taste, texture and appearance, along with conferring on them a wide range of health benefits, some of which are central to maintaining gut health and, in turn, mental health. These benefits are as follows:

1. Enhancing Microbial Diversity

Consuming fermented foods introduces a variety of beneficial microbes to the gut, increasing its microbial diversity. Diverse gut microbiota are associated with better resilience against infections, improved digestion and overall health.

2. Improving Digestion and Cleansing the Colon

A high concentration of probiotics and the production of certain organic acids through fermentation assist the stomach in digesting food more effectively. Additionally, they let the entirety of the undigested food pass through the small intestine smoothly, to be collected by the colon.

3. Boosting Emotional Well-Being

Numerous prebiotic ingredients are used while making fermented products. Ingredients like garlic, ginger, lemongrass, cabbage, onions, mustard seeds, and such others have a direct effect on regulating mood, reducing stress and anxiety, and promoting overall emotional well-being.

4. Removing Toxins from the Body

The high probiotic content of fermented foods protects the intestinal barrier and prevents the leakage of pathogens and heavy metal toxins such as lead, arsenic and cadmium into the bloodstream. Instead, a stable gut lining ensures the excretion of these toxins from the body via the colon.

5. Improving Cognition and Brain Functionality

Substances present in fermented foods stimulate the production of bioactive peptides exhibiting neuroprotective effects. They also stimulate the secretion of BDNF, which serves as a neurotransmitter modulator essential for learning, comprehension and memory.

All the additives and the core ingredients used for making fermented foods serve as a rich source of vitamins and other micronutrients like zinc, sodium, iron, and so on.

Reclaiming Your Identity and Health

Remember 'Manoj', the man with the identity crisis and poor self-esteem? First, his sedentary lifestyle led to obesity. Then excessive drinking and emotional eating compounded his struggles with weight gain and self-image, culminating in an identity crisis. The man who once revelled in the company of friends now avoided social gatherings out of shame for what he had become. As indicated by his blood tests which we discussed earlier, he was suffering from leaky gut syndrome with significant micronutrient deficiencies. He was under both physiological and psychological stress. It became evident that Manoj's physical and mental health were intricately linked, and his treatment plan needed to address both aspects simultaneously.

Following a Holistic Approach to Healing

The cornerstone of Manoj's recovery was a strict lifestyle overhaul, centred on nurturing both his body and his mind. The treatment plan I devised was comprehensive, targeting his gut health, nutritional deficiencies and mental well-being.

1. **Dietary Interventions**

    - **Low-Carb/High-Fat Diet:** Manoj was put on a low-carb/high-fat diet to reduce inflammation and promote weight loss. This diet focused on whole, nutrient-dense foods, primarily consisting of vegetables, healthy fats and lean proteins.
    - **Home-Cooked Meals:** Manoj was encouraged to eat home-cooked meals rich in garlic and onions, both of which are known for their anti-inflammatory and prebiotic properties. He was asked to include asparagus and leeks—which support gut health—in his diet.
    - **Ginger Tea with Fennel Seeds:** I recommended that Manoj have ginger tea with fennel seeds in the evening. This soothing tea helps with digestion, reduces bloating and has anti-inflammatory effects.
    - **Incorporating Specific Recipes:** I provided him with recipes that included apples, barley and dandelion greens, which he was encouraged to include in his diet due to their beneficial effects on gut health. One such recipe was a warm barley and apple salad with dandelion greens, tossed in a light vinaigrette made from olive oil and lemon juice.

2. **Incorporation of Fermented Foods**

    - Manoj was introduced to homemade fermented foods like kefir and kimchi—which are rich in probiotics. These foods played a crucial role in restoring the balance of beneficial bacteria in his gut, improving his digestion and enhancing his mental health.

3. **Supplementation**

    - To address his micronutrient deficiencies, Manoj was put on a regimen of targeted supplements, including vitamin D, magnesium, zinc and B vitamins. These supplements were crucial in reducing inflammation, supporting cognitive function and improving overall health.

4. **Lifestyle Modifications**

    - **Social Interaction with Boundaries:** While Manoj was encouraged to reconnect with his social circle, he was strictly advised to avoid alcohol. This allowed him to enjoy the company of friends without falling back into old, destructive habits.
    - **Caffeine Elimination:** Manoj was also advised to stop consuming caffeine which could exacerbate anxiety, disrupt sleep patterns and potentially hinder his recovery.

Results: A Remarkable Transformation

Three months into the treatment, the changes in Manoj were nothing short of miraculous. His CRP levels were significantly reduced, indicating a dramatic decrease in systemic inflammation. More importantly, his serum zonulin levels decreased markedly, confirming the reversal of his leaky gut syndrome. As a cherry on the cake, he also lost 15 kg of body fat that improved his muscle tone. These physiological improvements were paralleled by a profound shift in his mental state.

Manoj's self-confidence and self-esteem witnessed a significant boost. The once-tormented man who avoided mirrors now carried himself with renewed pride. His mental health improved to the extent that he became self-motivated and resumed his responsibilities, including managing his family business. The emotional eating episodes that once plagued him became a thing of the past, replaced by mindful eating and a newfound appreciation for healthy, nutritious foods.

Manoj also rekindled old friendships and built new relationships. His social life flourished as he no longer felt ashamed of his appearance. Instead, he embraced the journey of self-improvement with vigour, transforming not just his body but his mind and spirit as well.

The Renaissance

Manoj's journey is a testament to the power of holistic healing. It was not just about shedding pounds or managing symptoms; it was about reclaiming his identity and rediscovering the person he lost somewhere along the way. The dietary changes, lifestyle modifications and supportive therapies helped him rebuild his self-image and restore his health.

This transformation was not simply a physical one; it was an awakening. Manoj emerged from the depths of despair with a newfound zest for life, no longer shackled by self-doubt or poor health. He became a beacon of resilience, demonstrating that with the right guidance and determination, one could truly reinvent oneself.

As I reflect on his journey, I am filled with pride and admiration for the man who once stood before me, broken and lost. Today, Manoj is not just a man who overcame obesity and a poor self-image, he is a man reborn—living proof that the path to wellness is one of courage, perseverance and unwavering commitment to oneself.

Look No Far but within Your Home

Primary examples of fermented foods and beverages include yogurt, pickles, bread, kefir, beers, kimchi, sauerkraut, kombucha and wines. And here is the good part—instead of buying industrially made fermented food products, you can make many of these foods at home by yourself. There are compelling reasons to embrace the tradition of making these fermented foods at home. The process not only offers numerous health benefits but also fosters a deeper connection to what we consume. Here's why you should consider preparing these probiotic-rich foods in your own kitchen.

1. Superior Health Benefits

When you make fermented foods at home, you have complete control over the ingredients and the fermentation process, ensuring the highest quality and potency of probiotics. Commercially produced fermented products often undergo pasteurization which can kill beneficial bacteria. Additionally, they may contain additives, preservatives and high levels of sugar which can undermine their health benefits. By crafting your own food, you ensure that you're consuming the freshest, most potent probiotics available.

2. Economic and Environmental Benefits

Producing fermented foods at home is remarkably cost-effective. The ingredients required for fermentation—such as milk for yogurt, cabbage for sauerkraut and kimchi, and tea and sugar for kombucha—are inexpensive and readily available. Over time, the savings compared to purchasing commercial products can be significant.

Moreover, homemade fermentation is an environmentally friendly practice. It reduces your reliance on single-use packaging which is ubiquitous in store-bought products, and minimizes the carbon footprint associated with industrial production and transportation. By fermenting at home, you contribute to a more sustainable food system.

3. Culinary Creativity and Customization

Fermenting foods at home opens up a world of culinary creativity. You can experiment with different flavours, textures and ingredients to suit your personal taste preferences. For instance, when making yogurt, you can choose your preferred type of milk—be it cow's milk, goat's milk or plant-based alternatives—and adjust the fermentation time to achieve the desired consistency and tanginess.

Similarly, kimchi and sauerkraut recipes can be customized with various vegetables, spices and seasoning levels to create unique flavour profiles. Kombucha enthusiasts can explore an array of tea bases and flavour infusions, resulting in a personalized and ever-evolving beverage selection. This customization not only enhances your enjoyment of fermented foods but also ensures that they fit seamlessly into your diet and lifestyle.

Preparations and Recipes

Having learnt about all the benefits of probiotics and why we should prefer making them at home, let's look at the recipes of some probiotic-rich fermented foods and beverages that are easy to make.

1. **Kimchi:** Kimchi is a traditional Korean dish made by fermenting vegetables with a variety of seasonings. The most common type of kimchi is made with napa cabbage (aka

Chinese cabbage), but it can also include other vegetables such as radishes, green onions and cucumbers. The vegetables are typically mixed with ingredients like garlic, ginger, red chili flakes, fish sauce and salt. This mixture is then left to ferment at room temperature before being stored in the refrigerator.

Ingredients

- 1 large napa cabbage (about 2 pounds)
- ¼ cup sea salt
- 2 cups water
- 1 tablespoon grated ginger
- 5 cloves garlic, minced
- 1 tablespoon sugar
- 3 tablespoons red chili flakes
- 4 green onions, chopped
- 1 medium carrot, julienned[30]
- 1 daikon radish, julienned (optional)
- 2 tablespoons fish sauce or soy sauce (optional for vegan version)

Recipe Instructions

1. Prepare the cabbage
    - Cut the napa cabbage lengthwise into quarters and then into bite-sized pieces.
    - In a large bowl, dissolve the sea salt in the water. Add the cabbage and let it soak for 1–2 hours, tossing occasionally to ensure even salting.

---

[30]Julienne: It refers to a technique used to prepare vegetables by cutting them into matchstick-shaped pieces.

2. Rinse and drain
   - Rinse the cabbage thoroughly under cold water to remove excess salt. Drain well and squeeze out any remaining water.
3. Make the kimchi paste
   - In a small bowl, mix the ginger, garlic, sugar and red chili flakes. Adjust the amount of red chili flakes according to your desired spice level.
   - Add the fish sauce or soy sauce (if using), and mix well to form a paste.
4. Combine vegetables and paste
   - In a large mixing bowl, combine the drained cabbage, green onions, carrot and daikon radish (if using).
   - Add the kimchi paste and mix thoroughly, using your hands to ensure the vegetables are evenly coated. Wearing gloves is recommended to protect your skin from the chili pepper.
5. Pack the kimchi
   - Pack the mixture tightly into a clean, sterilized jar, pressing down to remove any air bubbles. Leave some space at the top to allow it to expand during fermentation.
6. Fermentation
   - Seal the jar and let it sit at room temperature for 1–5 days, depending on the ambient temperature and your taste preference. Check daily and press down the vegetables to keep them submerged in the brine.
   - Taste the kimchi daily; once it reaches your desired level of fermentation, transfer the jar to the refrigerator. The kimchi will continue to ferment slowly and develop more complex flavours over time.

2. **Sauerkraut:** Sauerkraut, which translates to 'sour cabbage' in German, is made by fermenting finely shredded cabbage with salt. Originating from Central and Eastern Europe, sauerkraut is created through a simple process where the cabbage is massaged with salt until it releases enough liquid to form a brine. The cabbage is then packed tightly into a jar or crock and left to ferment at room temperature.

Ingredients:

- 1 medium green cabbage (about 2 pounds)
- 1 tablespoon sea salt
- 1 tablespoon caraway seeds (optional)
- 1 teaspoon juniper berries (optional)

Recipe Instructions

1. Prepare the cabbage
   - Remove the outer leaves of the cabbage and set aside. Cut the cabbage into quarters, remove the core and finely shred it using a knife or a mandoline.
2. Mix with salt
   - In a large mixing bowl, combine the shredded cabbage with sea salt. Let it sit for 10 minutes to draw out moisture, then massage the cabbage vigorously with your hands until it releases enough liquid to create a brine (about 5–10 minutes).
3. Add flavourings
   - Add the caraway seeds and juniper berries (if using) to the cabbage and mix well.
4. Pack the cabbage
   - Pack the cabbage tightly into a clean, sterilized jar or fermentation crock, pressing down firmly to ensure the

cabbage is submerged in its own brine. Use the outer leaves to help keep the shredded cabbage submerged.
5. Fermentation
   - Place a weight on top of the cabbage to keep it submerged. Cover the jar with a cloth or fermentation lid to allow gases to escape while keeping contaminants out.
   - Let the sauerkraut ferment at room temperature for 1–4 weeks, depending on your taste preference and the ambient temperature. Check regularly and press down the cabbage if needed, to keep it submerged.
6. Storage
   - Once the sauerkraut has reached your desired level of tanginess, transfer it to the refrigerator. It will continue to develop flavour slowly and can be stored for several months.

3. **Kefir:** Kefir is a creamy, slightly fizzy fermented beverage that can be made from dairy milk (cow, goat or sheep) or non-dairy alternatives (such as coconut milk, almond milk or water). Originating from the Caucasus region, kefir is traditionally made by fermenting milk with kefir grains, which are not true grains but symbiotic cultures of bacteria and yeast (SCOBY). These grains ferment the sugars in the milk, producing a beverage rich in beneficial probiotics, vitamins and minerals. Of note, kefir grains are a combination of lactic acid bacteria, yeasts and polysaccharides. Known for its tangy flavour, this probiotic-rich drink has been celebrated for its ability to support gut health, boost the immune system, and provide a wealth of nutrients. Let's explore how to prepare kefir at home, along with a simple recipe to get you started.

Ingredients

- 1–2 tablespoons of kefir grains
- 4 cups of milk (dairy or non-dairy)
- A clean glass jar
- A plastic or wooden spoon
- A fine mesh strainer (plastic or stainless steel)

Recipe Instructions

1. Gather your ingredients and equipment
   - Ensure that all your equipment is clean to prevent contamination. Avoid using metal utensils as they can react with the kefir grains.
2. Combine the kefir grains and milk
   - Place the kefir grains in the clean glass jar. Pour the milk over the grains, leaving about an inch of space at the top of the jar to allow for expansion during fermentation.
3. Cover and ferment
   - Cover the jar with a cloth or a coffee filter, and secure it with a rubber band. This allows the kefir to breathe while keeping contaminants out.
   - Place the jar in a warm, dark place (ideally between 65°F and 85°F) and let it ferment for 24–48 hours. The fermentation time can be adjusted based on your taste preference—the longer it ferments, the tangier and thicker the kefir will become.
4. Strain the kefir
   - After the fermentation period, strain the kefir into a bowl using the fine mesh strainer. Use a plastic or wooden spoon to gently stir and help the liquid pass through, leaving the grains behind in the strainer.

5. Store the kefir
   - Transfer the strained kefir into a clean jar or bottle and store it in the refrigerator. It will continue to ferment slowly in the fridge and develop more complex flavours over time. Kefir can be consumed immediately or chilled for obtaining a refreshing drink.
6. Reuse the grains
   - Place the kefir grains back into the original jar and add fresh milk to start a new batch. Kefir grains can be reused indefinitely if properly cared for.

Tips for Making the Perfect Kefir

- **Adjust Fermentation Time:** Taste your kefir periodically to find the fermentation time that best suits your palate. A shorter fermentation time results in a milder flavour, while longer fermentation time creates a tangier taste.
- **Experiment with Flavours:** After straining, you can add flavours to your kefir by mixing in fruit, honey, vanilla extract or other natural flavourings.
- **Use High-Quality Ingredients:** Opt for high-quality milk (organic or raw if possible) to ensure the best taste and nutritional profile.

Keep in Mind

Incorporating prebiotic-rich foods into your diet can have numerous benefits for both your gut and mental health. By fostering a healthy gut microbiome, prebiotics can enhance digestive health, boost the immune system, and support mental well-being, including improved mood, cognitive function and stress response. A variety of prebiotic foods such as chicory root, garlic, onions and bananas can be a simple and effective way to promote overall health.

While stress affects our gut health, we can also focus on our gut health as a way to reduce stress. We can increase the number of beneficial bacteria in our gut by consuming probiotic-rich foods or taking probiotic supplements. Some of these bacteria produce neurotransmitters such as serotonin and GABA, and by maintaining a healthy balance of good bacteria in the gut, we can support our mental health and reduce stress levels. By supporting the gut barrier through the consumption of prebiotic-rich foods such as fibre, we can reduce inflammation and the impact of stress on the gut.

Inulin, FOS and GOS are powerful prebiotics that promote gut health by fostering the growth of beneficial bacteria and producing SCFAs during fermentation. SCFAs play a pivotal role in maintaining gut integrity, reducing inflammation and supporting overall gut health. Moreover, through the gut-brain axis, SCFAs influence neurotransmitter production and mitigate systemic inflammation, thereby contributing to improved mental health. Understanding these mechanisms highlights the importance of incorporating prebiotics into the diet for both the gut and mental well-being.

Fermented products like yogurt, kimchi, sauerkraut and kombucha are more than just flavourful additions to our diet. They are powerful probiotics that enhance gut health through various mechanisms, including improving microbial diversity, competing with pathogens, producing antimicrobial substances, modulating the immune system, strengthening the gut barrier, and providing metabolic benefits. Embracing these traditional foods can lead to a healthier gut and, by extension, a healthier life.

6

Nourishing the Brain: Foods That Support Neurotransmitters

In the grand tapestry of health, the threads of diet, gut microbiota and mental well-being are inextricably woven together. Foods rich in amino acids, neurotransmitters and micronutrients provide the essential substrates for neurotransmitter synthesis, and support a robust gut microbiome. This symbiotic relationship underpins the intricate dialogue between our gut and brain, shaping our mood, cognition and overall mental health. As we embrace the burgeoning science of nutritional psychiatry, it becomes abundantly clear that the pathway to a sound mind begins in the gut.

When 'Sarah' came to me with her loneliness and anger issues, she was experiencing persistent feelings of sadness, low energy, and a lack of interest in activities she once enjoyed. She found it challenging to concentrate at work and was withdrawing from social interactions. We diagnosed her with major depressive disorder.

As Sarah's nutritionist, I recognized the potential benefits of a nutritional intervention alongside traditional therapy. We took a holistic approach to managing her depression. I worked closely with her psychiatrist to carefully taper down her anti-anxiety pills and antidepressants. Along with therapy sessions and medication, Sarah's treatment plan included dietary changes and targeted nutritional supplementation, which included foods rich in omega-3 fatty acids, vitamin B12 and folate, and supplements containing vitamin D3 and NAD+.[31] Since zinc plays a crucial role in neurotransmitter function and mood regulation, a zinc supplement was also added to her regime.

I encouraged her to consume fatty fish (which are also good sources of NAD+) such as salmon, mackerel and sardines at least twice a week. Additionally, she included sources of plant-based omega-3s, such as flaxseeds, chia seeds and walnuts, in her meals. Vitamin D is essential for serotonin production and its daily intake helped alleviate Sarah's depressive symptoms. Folic acid, a B vitamin, is known to support neurotransmitter synthesis and regulate mood. I included folate-rich foods like leafy green vegetables, beans and fortified grains in her meals. Additionally, Sarah was advised to take a folic acid supplement to ensure optimal levels.

I closely monitored Sarah's progress, including regular check-ins with her therapist and her food intake. She kept a food diary to track her dietary intake and adherence to the nutritional recommendations. Any concerns or changes in symptoms were addressed promptly, and adjustments to the treatment plan were made as needed.

Over six weeks, Sarah completely came off her medications as she began to notice improvements in her mood and energy levels. She became more outgoing and reported feeling more

---

[31] Nicotinamide adenine dinucleotide (NAD+): It is a non-protein compound that serves as a catalyst and a mediator for multiple metabolic pathways and cellular processes central to DNA repair, energy production and immune function. It has also been found to improve cognitive function—including memory, focus and concentration.

engaged in activities, sleeping better, and experiencing fewer intrusive negative thoughts. It took another six weeks with the combined approach of therapy and nutritional intervention for her symptoms of depression to gradually resolve, allowing her to regain a sense of control and well-being in her life.

Sarah's case exemplifies the potential benefits of integrating nutritional intervention into the treatment of depression. By addressing potential nutrient deficiencies and incorporating foods and supplements rich in omega-3 fatty acids, zinc, vitamin D3, folic acid and NAD+ alongside counselling therapy, individuals like Sarah can optimize their mental health outcomes, and benefit from a holistic approach to wellness. It also underscores the importance of personalized and comprehensive care in managing depression and promoting overall well-being.

Fire up Your Neurons with Food

Food can affect mood. Importantly, the reverse is true as well. We discussed 'the dopamine connection to processed foods' in Chapter 2 and how stress alters our eating behaviour in Chapter 3—establishing that the state of our mind influences our eating habits. Individuals with a positive state of mind tend to make healthier food choices as they consider the future health benefits thereof. Conversely, people who are feeling low focus more on indulgence as they seek comfort or pleasure from the outside world which they cannot achieve from the inside. Unfortunately, what they usually find first is junk or packaged foods which are readily available. These are often crunchy and rich in salt or sugar, giving them the ability to trigger a 'dopamine rush', and a sense of reward to invoke feelings of pleasure and satisfaction later. However, this satisfaction is temporary and after some time, the brain and mind want more.

What we eat is what we think, and how and what we think are what we eat—this becomes a feedback cycle.

At this point in time, a mental health patient needs to make a conscious choice to get out of this vicious loop, and make a constant effort to eat healthy. The first aspect of treating mental health through the gut involves increasing the availability of neurotransmitters and their precursor molecules. Also, it involves creating an environment conducive to the production and working of neurotransmitters, which is where gut health actually comes into play.

Neurotransmitters, as previously discussed, mediate the electrochemical transmission between neurons, negotiating numerous functions critical for life, including emotional responses and the physical ability to feel pleasure and pain. Any imbalance in their levels can cause a range of neurological and psychiatric disorders—from Parkinson's disease to depression and memory loss to anxiety. Hence, it is a no-brainer that naturally occurring foods offering neurotransmitters and/or their precursors are a potential alternative to help prevent brain and psychiatric disorders.

Neurotransmitters are synthesized from simple and widely available compounds like amino acids with few conversion steps.

By changing dietary habits and modifying nutritional regimens, we can influence neurotransmitter levels in a manner that can improve both mental health and overall well-being. Dietary changes and nutritional interventions are no longer a mere support to traditional therapy. Nutritionists and healthcare practitioners working with functional medicine—which places a significant emphasis on the role of food and nutritional intake in optimizing health and treating mental illness—continue to incorporate dietary changes offering beneficial outcomes on some mental health disorders such as anxiety, depression and bipolar disorder.

Most psychiatric patients opting for alternative medicine treatments take this route only after coming to the realization that their food choices could be a modulator of their mood. Food has indeed been identified to affect our mood on the basis of the availability of neurotransmitters and their precursors, and a healthy gut making effective and efficient use of them. In addition, nutritional supplements containing a blend of micronutrients could help patients recover from restlessness and depressive symptoms.

Neurotransmitters are present in both plant and animal-based food. Glutamate, acetylcholine (ACh), GABA, dopamines and serotonin are distributed evenly to occur naturally in some animal foods, fruits, edible plants and roots. So whether you are a pure vegetarian or only follow a carnivore diet, you need not worry as nature has a lot to offer in both cases.

Of note, every micronutrient and essential amino acid play a critical role in maintaining and promoting gut health, especially when a lot of them serve as food for good bacteria and exhibit antioxidant and anti-inflammatory properties. These micronutrients are also essential for neurotransmitter production or regulation in the gut and the brain. So before we even discuss food sources from which we can derive the maximum neurotransmitters, let's first look at micronutrients that can help improve our brain function and boost mental health.

Micronutrients Boosting Neurotransmitter Production

The availability of micronutrients is linked to emotional regulation and mental health as certain micronutrients play a critical role in metabolic pathways in the brain. The primary micronutrients essential for maintaining mental health are folic acid, vitamins D3, B6 and B12, iron, magnesium, selenium, and zinc. We list such micronutrients and their sources below, and describe their selected brain-related functions central to boosting the production of neurotransmitters, and thus improving mental health.

- **Vitamin D3**
  - Food sources: Fish (salmon and sardines), canned tuna, eggs, shrimp and mushrooms. Also available in products fortified with vitamin D, such as regular milk, almond milk, and unsweetened yogurt and oatmeal
  - Essential to the production of serotonin—regulates the mood and reduces depression and anxiety symptoms
  - Improves brain function as many of the vitamin D receptors are present in high concentrations on the neurons in the brain

- **Choline**
  - Food sources: Whole eggs, organ meat (liver and kidneys), caviar, fish (salmon, tuna and cod), soybean, cruciferous vegetables (like cauliflower and broccoli) and almonds
  - Critical to the production of acetylcholine
  - Upregulates gene expressions involved in neuronal communication (neurotransmission)
  - During pregnancy, an expecting mother must ensure the intake of an optimal amount of choline to prevent her child from developing schizophrenia and other mental illnesses later in life.

B vitamins like B6, B12 and folate are vital for converting amino acids into neurotransmitters. They also support the production of DNA and the maintenance of nerve cells.

> **Folate (Vitamin B9)**

- Food sources: Leafy vegetables (spinach and kale), cruciferous vegetables (broccoli and cabbage), citrus fruits, avocado, eggs, beef and whole grains
- One of the essential vitamins (B9) to be sourced from our diet as our body cannot make it, and it can only be consumed through foods in the form of folate
- Folic acid is the synthetic form of folate added in supplements, bread, flour and ready-to-eat foods
- Upregulates the expression of BDNF, preventing 'leaky brain' and neuroinflammation, thus maintaining mental health
- Critical for the functioning of those enzymes that convert tryptophan into serotonin
- Crucial for those enzymes converting tyrosine into norepinephrine or noradrenalin
- Multiple studies have indicated the use of folate-rich foods and folic acid supplements to reduce symptoms of depression (postpartum and major), schizophrenia and bipolar disorders.[32] [33]

---

[32]Sakuma, K., et al., 'Folic acid/methylfolate for the treatment of psychopathology in schizophrenia: a systematic review and meta-analysis', *Psychopharmacology (Berl)*, Vol. 235, No. 8, 2018, pp. 2303–14.

[33]Nelson, S.L., et al., 'The potential use of folate and its derivatives in treating psychiatric disorders: A systematic review', *Biomedicine & Pharmacotherapy*, Vol. 146, 2022, p. 146.

Folic Acid + Vitamin B12 → Methionine → SAM → Serotonin and Dopamine Dopamine → Norepinephrine[34]

- **Vitamin B12**
  - Food sources: Mushrooms, kidney beans, yogurt, tofu, cheese, fish (trout, sardines, salmon, tuna), eggs, organ meat (liver), red meat (ground beef) and nutritional yeast
  - Involved in maintaining neural connections and normal nerve conductance for smooth signalling, thereby strengthening the gut-brain axis
  - Plays an important role in the metabolism of folate and many amino acids that are metabolized for the synthesis of neurotransmitters
  - Critical for the production of SAM (S-adenosylmethionine), a molecule that the body requires for synthesizing multiple neurotransmitters like norepinephrine, dopamine and serotonin

- **Vitamin B6**
  - Food sources: Avocado, garlic, ginger, onions, chickpeas, milk, tofu, salmon, tuna, eggs, bananas and pistachio
  - Plays an important role in the metabolism of folate to produce methionine and SAM, thus contributing to the production of serotonin, dopamine and norepinephrine

---

[34]Metabolic steps are only a representation of a very large cycle involving amino acids and vitamins to produce, recycle and use neurotransmitters. These do not indicate the actual metabolism.

- Critical for the efficient functioning of enzymes involved in the production of serotonin and dopamine. Serotonin has been indirectly found to support the synthesis of oxytocin. Hence, B6 also becomes important for the production of oxytocin in the brain.
- It is also important for enzymes participating in converting glutamate to GABA.
- Furthermore, it boosts the production of endorphins.

> **Vitamin B1**

- Food sources: Salmon, legumes (green peas, lentils and kidney beans), organ meat (liver), almonds, sunflower seeds, yogurt, wholegrain bread, fortified cereals
- Serves as a cofactor[35] for enzymes involved in the synthesis of acetylcholine. In simpler words, enzymes involved in the metabolism process to synthesize acetylcholine cannot function efficiently without vitamin B1
- Functions as a substitute for acetylcholine as it mimics its action in the brain
- Helps reduce mental fatigue, frustration and agitation

> **Vitamin B2**

- Food sources: Milk, yogurt, cheese, tofu, eggs, beef, pork, chicken breast, organ meat (beef liver), salmon,

---

[35] A cofactor is a non-protein chemical compound or metallic ion that is required for an enzyme's role as a catalyst to carry out a metabolic reaction or step.

clams, oysters, mushrooms, spinach, almonds and avocados
- Improves brain function by boosting the metabolism of essential fatty acids in brain lipids
- Exhibits antioxidant properties in the brain and gut
- Plays an important role in methionine synthesis from homocysteine

Vitamin B3

- Food sources: Organ meat (liver), chicken breast, fish (salmon and tuna), peanuts, avocado, almonds, brown rice, whole wheat, mushrooms, green peas and potatoes
- It is incorporated in NAD+ which serves as a cofactor to enzymes involved in the synthesis of acetylcholine.

Vitamin B5

- Food sources: Broccoli, cauliflower, cabbage, kidney beans, green peas, chickpeas, mushrooms, eggs, peanuts and sunflower seeds
- Involved in the synthesis of GABA, serotonin and dopamine
- Contributes to the structure and function of brain cells

Vitamin E

- Food sources: Avocado, almonds, walnuts, hazelnuts, peanuts, sunflower seeds, wheat germ oil, salmon, kiwi, turnip greens, broccoli and spinach
- Assists immune function and suppresses neuroinflammation

- Acts as an antioxidant that protects cells from damage from free radicals, thereby preventing neurodegeneration

> **Vitamin C**

- Food sources: Garlic, ginger, onions, guavas, melons (cantaloupe and muskmelons), parsley, kale, kiwi, broccoli, Brussels sprouts, cucumber, lemons, strawberries and oranges
- Facilitates neurotransmission that leads to the production and release of glutamate in the brain
- Serves as a cofactor for the enzyme involved in synthesizing L-DOPA, which further gets converted to dopamine
- Important for the enzyme converting dopamine into noradrenaline
- Required for the production of endorphins
- Acts as an antioxidant that protects cells from damage done by free radicals, thereby preventing neurodegeneration

Phenylalanine → Tyrosine → L-DOPA → Dopamine → Norepinephrine

> **Calcium**

- Food sources: Milk (cow's milk, almond and soy milk), yogurt, tofu, cheese (cheddar, mozzarella, feta), leafy green vegetables (spinach, kale, collard greens), nuts and seeds (almonds, chia and sesame), fish (sardines and salmon) and millets (foxtail and finger)
- Important for the release of neurotransmitters and several forms of chemical signalling between

cells including the one involved in gut-brain communication

- **Magnesium**
  - Food sources: Legumes (black beans, chickpeas, lentils), whole grains (amaranth, brown rice, quinoa, oats, whole wheat), nuts and seeds (almonds, cashews, pumpkin seeds, flaxseeds, chia seeds), ginger, garlic, onion and tofu
  - Essential for over 300 enzymatic reactions, including those involved in neurotransmitter synthesis
  - Important for the active transportation of ions (such as potassium and calcium) across cell membranes, and cell signalling
  - It also supports muscle and nerve function, blood glucose control and bone health.

- **Zinc**
  - Food sources: Almonds, cashews, raisins, red meat (ground beef), pumpkin seeds, sesame seeds, beans, oysters and tofu
  - Essential for neurons and the functioning of glial cells that are important for developing memory and cognitive function
  - Upregulates BDNF expression, thereby preventing leaky gut and neural inflammation
  - Strengthens synaptic plasticity, aiding in neurogenesis,[36] neuronal communication and signalling, and preventing pathological states

---

[36]Neurogenesis: It is the process by which new neurons are formed in the brain.

- Zinc deficiency has been linked to mood disorders and impaired cognitive function

> **Iron**

- Food sources: Amaranth, legumes (kidney beans, lentils and chickpeas), dark leafy green vegetables (spinach, silver beet and broccoli), red meat (ground beef), poultry (chicken and turkey), eggs, tofu, seafood (salmon, sardines and tuna), organ meat (liver and kidney), nuts (pistachios and munakka) and seeds (chia, pumpkin and sunflower)
- Essential cofactor for the production of energy in the brain
- Functions in the enzyme system involved in the production of neurotransmitters

> **Selenium**

- Food sources: Amaranth, nuts (cashews, Brazil nuts), seeds (chia, flaxseeds, sunflower), fish (trout, tuna), red meat (ground beef), tofu and eggs
- Forms a part of antioxidant enzymes that protect cells from damage by free radicals, thereby preventing neurodegeneration

Amino Acids as Building Blocks of the Neurotransmitters

Amino acids are the ***building blocks of proteins and the most crucial requirement*** for the production of neurotransmitters like serotonin, dopamine and norepinephrine, which play a critical role in mood regulation. For instance, the amino acid glutamine serves as a substrate for producing glutamate, the most abundant neurotransmitter in the body. Glutamate not only boosts certain brain functions but also serves as a precursor to producing GABA.

Whole foods such as leafy vegetables, lentils, lean meats, eggs, dairy products and tofu provide a rich source of protein and amino acids. Additionally, they are rich in micronutrients, and saturated and mono-saturated fats, promoting gut health. Conversely, industrially processed and sugar-rich foods throw off the balance within the gut microbiota in favour of pathogenic bacteria, resulting in their overgrowth and hindering the growth of beneficial bacteria.

We just discussed major micronutrients that support brain health and produce neurotransmitters, serving as key players in maintaining and enhancing mental health. Now we divert our attention to amino acids essential for the same. Amino acids can be categorized into two groups:

1. **Non-essential amino acids**: Those which can be synthesized by the body; for instance, alanine, cysteine, glutamic acid, *glutamine*, glycine, *tyrosine,* and so on
2. **Essential amino acids**: Those which cannot be synthesized in the body and must be obtained through diet or supplements; for instance, isoleucine, leucine, *methionine*, *phenylalanine*, *tryptophan*, valine, and so on

We will keep our focus on the amino acids marked in bold and italics as they are the ones directly or majorly involved in contributing to our mental health by either helping to produce neurotransmitters and promoting gut health, or boosting brain function by enhancing neuronal health.

> **Glutamic Acid or Glutamine**
>
> ♦ Food sources: Eggs, beef, fish (sardines, shrimps), seaweed, tofu, corn, red cabbage, soybean, red kidney

beans, dairy products (milk, cheese, yogurt) and nuts (almonds, walnuts, cashews). Note: Glutamic acid is naturally found in foods rich in protein.
- Serves as a fuel for enterocytes (intestinal cells), supporting the integrity of the gut lining and strengthening the barrier, thereby promoting nutrient absorption, preventing leaky gut and promoting gut health
- Boosts our overall immune function
- Serves as a substrate for producing glutamate which is further used to synthesize GABA

> **Tyrosine**

- Food sources: Beef, turkey, chicken breast, fish (salmon, tuna), tofu, dairy (cheese, milk), nuts and seeds (peanuts, cashews, pistachios, walnuts, almonds, sesame seeds, pumpkin seeds) and soybean
- Produces L-DOPA which acts as a substrate for producing dopamine, thus increasing dopamine availability
- Indirectly involved in synthesizing norepinephrine as some of the dopamine is used to produce norepinephrine
- Involved in maintaining and repairing neural connections to boost the communication between nerve cells, thereby strengthening the gut-brain axis
- Helps us function under stress
- Boosts the performance of working memory and executive function

Tyrosine is literally a food for your thought.

- **Phenylalanine**
  - Food sources: Legumes (lentils, kidney beans, chickpeas), soy products and tempeh, meat and eggs, fish (salmon, trout, tuna, shrimp), whole grains (wheat, barley, oats), nuts (peanuts, cashews, pistachios, almonds)
  - Indirectly involved in producing dopamine and norepinephrine by getting converted into tyrosine.
  - Involved in neurotransmission from the brain to the body's nerve cells, in turn strengthening the gut-brain axis
  - Improves working memory

Phenylalanine → Tyrosine → L-DOPA → Dopamine → Norepinephrine[37]

- **Methionine**
  - Food sources: Eggs, beef, tuna, tofu, nuts and seeds (Brazil nuts, chia seeds, flaxseeds, cashews, pistachios), and legumes
  - Works with folic acid and vitamin B12 at critical steps for producing SAM (S-adenosylmethionine), a molecule that the body requires for synthesizing multiple neurotransmitters like norepinephrine, dopamine and serotonin

Folic Acid + Vitamin B12 → Methionine → SAM → Serotonin and Dopamine

---

[37]Metabolic steps are only a representation of a very large cycle involving amino acids and vitamins to produce, recycle and use neurotransmitters. These do not indicate the actual metabolism.

> **Tryptophan**
> - Food sources: Eggs, fish (salmon, sardines), dairy (cheese, milk), tofu, oatmeal, seeds (chia, pumpkin, sunflower seeds), vegetables (spinach, green peas, broccoli, soybean, kidney beans) and fruits (pineapple, kiwi, tomato)
> - Gets converted into serotonin, which helps regulate the mood and enhances cognitive functions
> - Gets converted into melatonin, which helps regulate the sleep-wake cycle

Tryptophan → 5-HT→ Serotonin → N-acetyleserotonin → Melatonin

---

Fine-Tuning GABA and Glutamate

Throughout the book, we have discussed the role of glutamate and GABA in managing various psychological and brain functions. Now if you noticed their roles, you would realize that they are the complete opposite of each other in terms of their mechanism of action. Where GABA is a calming messenger modulating stress responses by lowering anxiety, glutamate helps a person remain alert and active throughout the day, uplifting their mood by primarily keeping them motivated and excited. So both work to uplift the mood and modulate stress by taking different routes. GABA is an inhibitory neurotransmitter which works by inhibiting certain reactions or pathways in the brain. Conversely, glutamate is an excitatory neurotransmitter which works by triggering or exciting neurons to carry a message to the next set of neurons.

An optimally functional brain requires both excitatory and inhibitory inputs that are regulated and balanced. A perturbation

> in the excitatory/inhibitory balance leads to dysfunctional signalling, impairing cognitive and motor function, thus causing psychological and neurodevelopmental disorders. At the cellular level, the transmission of glutamate and GABA controls the excitatory/inhibitory balance and regulates the mood, which implies that it controls when one needs to remain alert or excited, and when to calm down and assess a situation. The good part is that the body's metabolic intelligence is such that it maintains a fine balance between synthesizing glutamate and using glutamate to produce GABA. However, when this balance is disrupted in case of a disease, one needs careful guidance from a nutritionist trying to treat a psychiatric issue through dietary intervention to maintain a fine balance between eating glutamate-rich and GABA-rich foods.

Omega-3s as a Facilitator of the Functioning of Neurotransmitters

As discussed in Part 1 of the book, omega-3 fatty acids are essential fatty acids that we need from our diet. The parent omega-3 is alpha-linolenic acid (ALA), and is further used to make eicosapentaenoic acid (EPA) and docosahexaenoic acid (DHA). However, due to poor conversion efficiency, physicians recommend consuming foods rich in EPA and DHA.

We discussed earlier in Part 1 how both omega-6 and omega-3 fatty acids are important but only in a said ratio—between 2:1 and 5:1—as large amounts of omega-6 have been linked to promoting inflammation. On the other hand, omega-3 fatty acids exhibit anti-inflammatory effects. Hence, it is recommended to increase the latter's presence in our diet.

In Pursuit of Happiness—Boosting Neural Health

Omega-3 fatty acids are the building blocks of brain cells. These fats bind to cell membranes, increasing fluidity which is important for the functioning of each brain cell, including adapting to a stressful situation and responding to a piece of new information. Additionally, the omega-3s in cell membranes aid in the functioning of neurotransmitter receptors, which help to:

- **Regulate the Mood**
  They increase the availability of serotonin—alleviating symptoms of depression and promoting a positive outlook at the time of distress. Also, they enhance the transmission of dopamine signals in the brain, contributing to improved motivation. Furthermore, they influence the release, and enhance the availability, of endorphins—natural pain-relieving and mood-elevating compounds which are crucial for our emotional well-being.
- **Improve Neurotransmission**
  They facilitate the overall communication of information in the brain.
- **Enhance Cognitive Function**
  DHA, in particular, is highly concentrated in the brain and is essential for cognitive functions, memory and learning. It supports neuroplasticity—the brain's ability to adapt and form new connections—which is crucial for learning and memory formation.
- **Reduce Neuroinflammation**
  Studies have shown that omega-3s increase the expression of our friend BDNF—the brain's growth hormone—thus increasing the production of brain messengers

while suppressing neuroinflammation.[38] These fats help produce anti-inflammatory metabolites in the brain that pose resistance to stress damage (like oxidative stress or hypoxia). EPA and DHA have neuroprotective properties, meaning they can help protect brain cells from damage and degeneration. This can potentially reduce the risk of age-related cognitive decline and neurodegenerative diseases like Alzheimer's and Parkinson's.

- **Improve Attention and Focus**
  Omega-3 fatty acids may also play a role in attention and focus, making them beneficial for individuals with ADHD or those seeking to enhance their cognitive performance.

Dietary Sources of Omega-3 Fatty Acids Include:

- Fish and other seafood (especially cold-water fatty fish such as salmon, mackerel, tuna, trout, sardines)
- Nuts and seeds (flaxseeds, chia seeds, walnuts)
- Plant oils (flaxseed oil)
- Fortified foods (certain brands of eggs, yogurt, juices, milk, soy beverages)

Jump through the Hoops—Eat Foods Rich in Neurotransmitters

Each neurotransmitter has its own assigned substrate—including many of the aforementioned nutrients—which should generally be included in the diet. However, plenty of foods naturally contain neurotransmitters, though data on their food sources

---

[38] Wu, A., Z. Ying, and F. Gomez-Pinilla, 'Dietary omega-3 fatty acids normalize BDNF levels, reduce oxidative damage, and counteract learning disability after traumatic brain injury in rats', *J Neurotrauma*, Vol. 21, No. 10, 2004, pp. 1457–67.

is insufficient *(which is where we have cut out the social media noise for you)*. So you can spare your liver from processing the substrate and metabolizing it via a well-defined pathway to form a neurotransmitter. Instead, you can directly take neurotransmitters by consuming certain foods as natural supplements. We will now discuss the nutritional associations and food sources of a few major neurotransmitters responsible for maintaining and boosting mental health, thereby highlighting the foods to be consumed for an effective intake of each neurotransmitter.[39][40]

Neurotransmitters	Food Sources
Serotonin	• Fruits—kiwi, cherries, green grapes, passionfruit, papaya, pineapple, plum, pomegranate, strawberries, tomato, bananas • Red pepper and paprika • Vegetables—cabbage, chicory (*kasni*), brinjal, legumes, onion and green onion, lettuce, potatoes • Oats, wild rice • Coffee • Velvet beans • Nuts (hazelnuts, walnuts) • Tryptophan-rich foods (see above)

---

[39] Gasmi, A., et al., 'Neurotransmitters Regulation and Food Intake: The Role of Dietary Sources in Neurotransmission', *Molecules*, Vol. 28, No. 1, 2022, p. 210.
[40] Briguglio, M., et al., 'Dietary Neurotransmitters: A Narrative Review on Current Knowledge', *Nutrients*, Vol. 10, No. 5, 2018, p. 591.

| Dopamine | - Velvet beans
- Meat, poultry, fish, eggs
- Dark chocolate, avocado, banana, apple, orange, tomato, watermelon
- French beans and kidney beans, peas, spinach
- Tyrosine and phenylalanine-rich foods (see above) |
|---|---|
| Glutamate | - Caviar, cheese, Parmesan cheese, tofu
- Mushrooms, fermented beans, soy sauces, vegetable soups, tomato, spinach
- Fish sauces, gravies, oyster sauce, seaweeds
- Coffee
- Meat, salami, eggs, beef, fish (sardines, cod, shrimp)
- Noodle, ready-to-eat meals, savoury snacks (in the form of monosodium glutamate)
- Red cabbage, soybean, red kidney beans
- Tomato, corn
- Dairy—milk, cheese, yogurt
- Nuts—almonds, walnuts, hazelnuts, cashews |

| GABA | - Green tea
- Fermented foods—kimchi, kefir, fermented beans, cheese, yogurt, fermented fish sauce
- Beans—lupin beans, soybeans, kidney beans, French beans, peas (its sprouted form is reported to have more GABA than its raw form)
- Other vegetables—broccoli, cabbage, cauliflower, spinach, potato, sweet potato, mushrooms
- Whole grains—oats, wheat, barley, wild rice, black rice, buckwheat (*kattu ka atta*)
- Chestnut, tomato
- Glutamic acid or glutamine-rich foods (see above)
- Glutamate-rich foods (see above) |
|---|---|
| Norepinephrine | - Bananas, beans, legumes
- Cheese
- Chicken, meat
- Fish—shrimp, halibut
- Oatmeal and chocolate
- Tyrosine-rich foods (see above) |
| Acetylcholine | - Squash (*chappan kaddu*), eggplant (brinjal), spinach
- French beans, soybeans, kidney beans, peas, radish
- Mistletoe (known for its sedative effects; also used in the treatment of headaches, hypertension and epilepsy)
- Bitter orange, wild strawberry
- Choline-rich foods (see above) |

Melatonin	- Nuts—pistachios, almonds, cashews
- Fruits—tart cherries, bananas, pineapples, red and black grapes
- Oats
- Fish—salmon and sardines
- Mushrooms
- Tryptophan and serotonin-rich foods (see above)
Oxytocin	- Dark chocolate
- Avocado and bananas
- Nuts and seeds—walnuts, chia seeds, flaxseeds
- Omega-3-rich foods—desi ghee, broccoli, cabbage
- Fish—salmon and sardines
- Tryptophan and serotonin-rich foods (see above), as serotonin has been found to indirectly support oxytocin production inside the brain
Endorphins	- Dark chocolate and cacao
- Fruits—strawberries and avocados
- Leafy greens—spinach, kale and Swiss chard
Histamines	- Fermented foods—sauerkraut, tempeh, fermented sausages
- Soy-based products—soy milk, soy sauce
- Aged cheeses—cheddar and Parmesan
- Fish—herring, sardines, tuna, mackerel and bonito

Additional Notes

- Acetylcholine, norepinephrine, serotonin and dopamine also enhance gastrointestinal motility, thereby preventing SIBO and promoting gut health.
- One additional amino acid—L-carnitine—supports brain function and serves as a natural anti-depressant. It acts through increasing quantities of norepinephrine and serotonin. It is primarily found in red meat, pork and chicken. Vegans can get it in smaller quantities through milk and hard cheese, but it is best for them to get it from L-carnitine supplements. One does not need more than 2 grams of L-carnitine a day, and it SHOULD NOT be considered for long-term use as it increases the risk of plaque build-up in the arteries, clogging them and causing atherosclerosis.
- ***A word of caution for potatoes and bananas***: While they are rich in neurotransmitters, they also contain high quantities of starch and simple carbohydrates—making them high glycemic-load foods which must be avoided to prevent hyperglycaemia, which results in diabetes (in the long run).
- ***More on velvet beans***: Also known as cowhage and *kaunch ke beej*, they have been used in herbal medications since ancient Ayurvedic times for the treatment of diabetes, stress and depression. They contain L-DOPA which is used as a precursor to synthesize dopamine. Due to this very reason, they have also been proved effective in treating Parkinson's disease. Also, velvet beans are rich in micronutrients like iron, magnesium and zinc—all of which play a crucial role in boosting brain function and maintaining mental health.

- ***Does dietary GABA actually reach the brain?*** It is debatable whether the oral intake of GABA can directly affect brain function. However, multiple studies have connected the actions of oral GABA to its effects on the enteric nervous system, which functions through the gut.[41] It has been confirmed in multiple studies that GABA crosses the blood-brain barrier only when needed. When one is unable to follow a mood-enhancing diet, nutritional supplementation with micronutrients like vitamins B, D, E, zinc, calcium and magnesium significantly ameliorates depressive symptoms and improves mental health. In addition, the consumption of omega-3 fatty acids and certain plant extracts may have an impact on mood balance.
- A promising biologically active plant substance—shown to reduce symptoms and help adapt to increased physical and emotional stress situations—is ashwagandha.

Restoring Gut Health and Mental Clarity

Remember the case we introduced in Chapter 3? When 'Emma' first walked into my office, it was evident that she was a woman carrying the weight of the world on her shoulders. At 38 years old, she was grappling with a myriad of physical and emotional challenges that slowly began to erode the quality of her life. A dedicated professional, Emma was always the kind of person who thrived under pressure, pouring her energy into her work to escape the stress and responsibilities that awaited her at home.

---

[41]Liwinski, T., et al., 'Exploring the Therapeutic Potential of Gamma-Aminobutyric Acid in Stress and Depressive Disorders through the Gut–Brain Axis, *Biomedicines*, Vol. 11, No. 12, 2023, p. 3128.

Given the clear connection between Emma's stress levels and her digestive issues, it was imperative to address both her physical symptoms and the underlying emotional stressors.

The Treatment Plan: A Path to Healing

I devised a comprehensive treatment plan focusing on dietary changes, lifestyle modifications and stress management techniques.

1. Dietary Interventions

- **Eliminating Caffeine and Alcohol:** The first step was to eliminate caffeine and alcohol from Emma's diet. Both substances can exacerbate stress and digestive issues, contributing to the vicious cycle of discomfort and anxiety she was experiencing.
- **A Diet Rich in Vegetables and Whole Grains:** To support her levels of serotonin and dopamine—critical neurotransmitters involved in mood regulation—I recommended a diet rich in vegetables like cabbage, chicory (kasni), brinjal, legumes, onion, green onion, lettuce, potatoes, velvet beans, French beans, kidney beans, peas and spinach. Not only are these foods nutrient-dense, they also support gut health and mental well-being.
- **Incorporating Nuts and Seeds:** For midday snacking, I encouraged Emma to include nuts and seeds like chia seeds, walnuts and almonds. These healthy fats provide sustained energy and support brain function.
- **Eliminating Wheat and Processed Foods:** Wheat was completely eliminated from Emma's diet, and I advised her to make rotis from whole grains like buckwheat and jowar millet. Processed foods such as bread, pizza, pasta

and cereals were also removed, along with high-glycemic foods like potatoes and rice.
- **Incorporating Fermented Foods:** To restore balance in her gut microbiome, I introduced fermented foods like kimchi, kefir, fermented beans, cheese, yogurt and fermented fish sauce into her diet. These foods are rich in probiotics which are essential for maintaining a healthy gut flora.
- **Healthy Cooking Oils:** I recommended that Emma avoid all vegetable oils except for coconut and olive oil, which have anti-inflammatory properties and support gut health.

2. **Stress Management and Lifestyle Changes**
   - Given the critical role that stress played in Emma's condition, I also encouraged her to adopt stress management techniques such as deep breathing exercises, mindfulness meditation and gentle physical activity like yoga or walking. These practices were designed to help her manage stress more effectively and reduce its impact on her digestive health.

Results: A Transformation in Mind and Body

Three months into the treatment, the results were remarkable. Emma's stress markers reduced to within acceptable levels, and her lactulose and mannitol test came back negative, indicating that her intestinal permeability was successfully treated. Her gut health improved significantly with her serum zonulin levels now within normal limits. Issues like abdominal discomfort, bloating and irregular bowel movements that plagued her for so long were largely resolved.

But the transformation extended far beyond the physical domain. Emma became a calmer, more centred person. The fatigue that once clouded her mind lifted, replaced by a newfound mental acuity and clarity. She reported feeling more cognitively sharp—she was able to think more clearly and make decisions with greater confidence.

This mental transformation had profound implications for her professional life. As a manager, Emma found that she could get more done in less time, and inspire and motivate her team more effectively. Her leadership qualities, once dulled by stress and fatigue, shone through with renewed brilliance. She became more proactive, taking on challenges with a sense of purpose and direction that eluded her before.

A Reflection on Emma's Journey

Emma's journey is a testament to the incredible resilience of the human body and spirit when given the right tools to heal. What began as a struggle with physical symptoms and emotional turmoil evolved into a profound transformation that touched every aspect of her life. Through a carefully tailored nutritional plan and lifestyle changes, Emma not only recovered her physical health but also reclaimed her mental clarity and self-confidence.

Her transformation into a new person—healed of her stressors—solidified my faith in the power of holistic healing. Emma's story is not just about overcoming bloating or fatigue, it is about rediscovering the strength within oneself to rise above challenges and emerge stronger, wiser and more fulfilled through nutritional and lifestyle changes. In the end, Emma didn't just regain her health—she found a new sense of self, a calmer mind and a sharper intellect.

Incorporating the Neuro-Friendly Plate in Your Meals

Understanding the significance of micronutrients and recognizing the nutritional profiles of wholesome foods is a great first step towards a healthier lifestyle. So let's take the next step by integrating these nutrient-packed foods into our daily meals. Below is a meal planner designed to help you incorporate foods rich in micronutrients and neurotransmitters in your breakfast, lunch, snacks and dinner.

Here are daily examples of how you can integrate simple yet effective practices into your routine to heal your gut and enhance your mental health:

Morning: Start Your Day with a Gut-Friendly Breakfast

Kick off your day with a nutrient-dense breakfast that supports gut health. A bowl of oatmeal topped with fresh berries, a spoonful of chia seeds and a dollop of yogurt is an excellent choice. The fibre in oatmeal aids digestion, while the probiotics in yogurt promote a healthy balance of gut bacteria. Additionally, berries are rich in antioxidants which help reduce inflammation in the gut. Furthermore, chia seeds provide omega-3 fatty acids and almonds add a good dose of vitamin E and magnesium.

Also, you can try a spinach and avocado smoothie which requires fresh spinach, avocado, banana, almond milk and a scoop of protein powder (optional). Spinach is packed with iron, magnesium and folate, along with a blend of neurotransmitters like glutamate, GABA and dopamine. Avocado provides healthy fats and potassium, whereas bananas boost serotonin levels and add potassium and vitamin B6.

Mid-Morning: Hydrate with Herbal Teas

Instead of reaching for a second cup of coffee, opt for herbal teas such as ginger, peppermint or chamomile. Ginger is loaded with prebiotics. These teas have soothing properties that can ease digestive discomfort and reduce stress levels. Staying hydrated is essential for maintaining a healthy digestive tract and herbal teas are a gentle way to keep your system running smoothly.

Lunch: Incorporate Fermented Foods

Make fermented foods a staple in your lunch. A salad with a side of kimchi or sauerkraut, or a sandwich with a spread of miso can significantly boost your intake of probiotics. These beneficial bacteria help maintain a healthy gut microbiome which is essential for nutrient absorption and mental well-being.

Afternoon: Mindful Snacking

Choose snacks that support gut health, such as a handful of almonds, a piece of fruit, or carrot sticks with hummus. These snacks are rich in fibre, vitamins and minerals, promoting a balanced digestive system. Avoid sugary or processed snacks which can disrupt the gut flora and lead to energy crashes and mood swings.

Evening: A Balanced Dinner with Prebiotics

For dinner, focus on a balanced meal that includes prebiotic-rich foods. Foods like garlic, onions, asparagus and bananas are excellent sources of prebiotics. A dinner of grilled salmon with a side of roasted asparagus and quinoa provides a perfect mix of nutrients to support gut and brain health.

Night: Wind Down with Relaxation Techniques

End your day with relaxation techniques that promote gut and mental health. Practices such as deep breathing exercises, meditation or gentle yoga can reduce stress and support healthy digestion. Stress is a major contributor to gut issues, and managing it effectively is crucial for both your digestive and mental well-being.

By incorporating these daily habits into your routine, you can create a positive feedback loop that nurtures both your gut and your mind. Remember, healing your gut is a journey that requires consistency and mindfulness, but the benefits of improved mental clarity, mood stability and overall health are well worth the effort.

Keep in Mind

By nurturing a balanced gut environment through lifestyle interventions, you can optimize your overall well-being and cultivate a symbiotic relationship between the gut and the brain. Embracing this holistic perspective paves the way for a healthier and more integrated approach to healthcare in the modern world.

By consuming anti-inflammatory foods rich in micronutrients and amino acids such as wholesome green vegetables, berries, whole grains and fatty fish, we can reduce inflammation and promote gut health. Micronutrients and amino acids support and enhance gut microbial diversity, ensuring a greater variety of beneficial bacteria found in the gut. A more diverse gut microbiome is considered to be healthier. The links and mechanisms that are found (the way the gut affects neurotransmitter production) may, in the future, allow for the earlier detection of diseases and their targeted treatment.

With each mindful bite, we not only nourish our bodies but also cultivate the very essence of our mental well-being. Let us embark on this gastronomic journey where every meal is a step towards holistic health, and every nutrient a catalyst for harmony and vitality. In this epicurean symphony, the gut and the mind perform a melodious duet, echoing the timeless truth: we are indeed what we eat.

7

The Elimination Protocol: A Path to Optimal Health

In the vast realm of nutrition, few approaches are as transformative and enlightening as the elimination protocol. This method isn't just a dietary regimen, it's a journey toward discovering the intricate relationship between what we consume and our overall well-being. The elimination protocol is a dietary strategy designed to identify and remove foods that may cause adverse reactions in the body. These reactions can manifest as digestive issues, skin problems, respiratory symptoms or general inflammation. By temporarily eliminating these potential triggers and then gradually reintroducing them, individuals can pinpoint specific food sensitivities or allergies.

When Is the Elimination Protocol Used?

The elimination protocol is particularly useful for individuals experiencing unexplained symptoms that may be linked to their diet. It has been commonly employed in cases of:

- **Food Allergies and Intolerances:** When specific foods cause immune responses or digestive discomfort
- **Autoimmune Diseases:** Conditions like Hashimoto's thyroiditis, rheumatoid arthritis and lupus, where dietary triggers may exacerbate symptoms

- **Chronic Inflammation:** Persistent inflammation that might be fuelled by certain dietary components
- **Digestive Disorders:** Issues such as irritable bowel syndrome (IBS), bloating, gas and other gastrointestinal disturbances

However, its use is now not limited to the fight against the above-mentioned disorders. It is now being recognized for its potential in managing mental health issues such as depression, bipolar disorder and anxiety. This dietary approach—involving the systematic removal and reintroduction of specific foods—has shown promise in alleviating symptoms and improving overall mental well-being.

How Does the Elimination Protocol Impact Mental Health?

1. Reducing Inflammation

As we understand the gut-brain axis and highlight the significant role of gut health in regulating mood, cognition and behaviour, it is easy to link certain foods causing inflammation (in the gut or in the brain) with poor mental health. Chronic inflammation is a common underlying factor in many mental health conditions. Inflammatory cytokines—signalling molecules of the immune system—can cross the blood-brain barrier and influence brain function. By reducing the dietary triggers of inflammation and gut dysbiosis, the elimination protocol can help manage symptoms of mental disorders including depression and anxiety.

2. Improving Gut Health

By eliminating foods that disrupt the gut microbiota and incorporating probiotics from fermented foods, the elimination protocol supports a healthy gut environment. A balanced gut microbiome is essential for producing neurotransmitters like serotonin which regulate the mood and anxiety.

3. Stabilizing Blood Sugar Levels

Removing processed foods and refined sugars helps stabilize blood sugar levels, which can have a profound impact on our mood and energy. Fluctuations in blood sugar are linked to mood swings, irritability and anxiety.

4. Enhancing Nutrient Intake

Adding whole, nutritionally dense foods ensures the adequate intake of vitamins, minerals and antioxidants that are crucial for brain health. Nutrient deficiencies are often linked to mental health disorders.

A systematic review published in *Public Health Nutrition* analyzed the effects of various dietary interventions on anxiety. The review highlighted several studies where eliminating common allergens and inflammatory foods resulted in a reduction in anxiety symptoms. The findings suggested that by targeting the dietary triggers of inflammation and gut dysbiosis, the elimination protocol can be an effective strategy for managing anxiety.[42] Additionally, research published in *The Journal of Clinical Psychiatry* explored the role of diet in managing bipolar disorder. The study found that patients with bipolar disorder often had comorbid conditions such as gastrointestinal issues and food sensitivities. Implementing the elimination protocol helped reduce mood swings and stabilize mental health by addressing

---

[42]Lee, M., and H. Lee, 'The Effect of Dietary Interventions on Mental Health Disorders: A Systematic Review', *Public Health Nutrition*, Vol. 18, No. 5, 2015, pp. 823–35.

these underlying dietary triggers.[43]

A Practical Guide to the Elimination Protocol to Enhance Mental Health

Phase I. Elimination

> **Eliminating Wheat and Corn Products**
>
> Wheat and corn are ubiquitous in modern diets, often found in bread, cookies, pasta, *chapati*s, noodles, sago, oats, semolina and corn-based foods. The first step in the elimination protocol is to remove these items from the diet.

Alternatives to Wheat and Corn

- **Millets**
  - **Besan (chickpea flour):** A versatile flour used in baking and cooking
  - **Ragi (finger millet):** Rich in calcium and fibre, perfect for porridge and flatbreads
  - **Jowar (sorghum):** Excellent for making roti and porridge
  - **Bajra (pearl millet):** Nutritious and suitable for flatbreads and porridge
  - **Amaranth:** A pseudo-grain high in protein and essential amino acids
  - **Buckwheat (kuttu ka atta):** Gluten-free and ideal for pancakes, noodles and baking
  - **Quinoa:** High in protein and fibre, perfect for salads and as a rice substitute

---

[43]Clayton, A., et al., 'Dietary Patterns and Bipolar Disorder: A Review of the Evidence', *The Journal of Clinical Psychiatry*, Vol. 74, No. 2, pp. 190–98.

- **Rolled Unprocessed Oats:** Suitable for making oatmeal and granola, ensuring that they are gluten-free

Eliminating Dairy Products

Dairy products including heavy cream, hard cheese, mozzarella and cottage cheese are common inflammation-causing foods that can cause digestive issues, skin problems and respiratory symptoms.

Alternatives to Dairy

- **Plant-Based Milks:** Almond milk, coconut milk, rice milk and oat milk
- **Non-Dairy Yogurts:** Coconut yogurt, almond yogurt and soy yogurt
- **Non-Dairy Cheeses:** Made from nuts like cashews or almonds, available in various flavours
- **Nutritional Yeast:** Provides a cheesy flavour and is rich in B vitamins

Eliminating Inflammatory Oils

- Refined oils such as sunflower, canola, safflower, rice bran, soybean, peanut and olive pomace oil can contribute to inflammation. These should be replaced with healthier options like:
  - **Extra-Virgin Olive Oil:** High in monounsaturated fats and antioxidants
  - **Coconut Oil:** Contains medium-chain triglycerides (MCTs) that provide quick energy
  - **Avocado Oil:** Rich in monounsaturated fats and suitable for cooking at high temperatures

- **Ghee (Clarified Butter):** Free of milk solids and suitable for those without a dairy sensitivity

Eliminating Sugars

- We eliminate white sugar along with honey, maple syrup and agave nectar.
- Very little sugar is allowed in its natural form such as organic jaggery, brown *khand* and stevia leaves.

Eliminating Processed Packaged Foods

Processed, packaged foods often contain preservatives, artificial additives, and high levels of sugar and unhealthy fats. These include cornflakes, muesli, chips and crackers, cookies, dips and sauces, tetrapack fruit juices, ready-to-eat food, instant soups and noodles, frozen food, mayonnaise and table butter.

Alternatives to Processed Foods

- **Whole Foods:** Fresh fruits, vegetables, whole grains, legumes, nuts and seeds
- **Homemade Snacks:** Vegetable sticks with hummus, homemade granola and fruit smoothies
- **Homemade Sauces and Dips:** Made from fresh ingredients without additives
- **Freshly Prepared Meals:** Cooking from scratch using whole food ingredients

Avoiding Fructose-Rich Fruits

- Fruits like red and golden apple, mango, grapes, banana, dates, figs, peach and melons need to be eliminated.

Alternative Fruits

- Berries: Strawberry, blueberry, cranberry, gooseberry, blackberry, *jamun*, *amla*
- Green apple (not more than half in a day), papaya (not more than one bowl)
- Avocado, olives, plums and fresh apricot

> **Avoiding Certain Animal Products**
>
> Fish, seafood and processed meats like sausage, ham, bacon and steak are eliminated due to potential allergens and additives. Fresh meat and clean eggs are acceptable alternatives (**only when dealing with mental health issues**). When we are trying to treat autoimmune disease, we eliminate meat and eggs of all kinds.

Alternatives to Processed Animal Products

- **Fresh Meat:** Such as chicken, beef, lamb and pork, after ensuring they are free from additives and preservatives
- **Clean Eggs:** From free-range or organic sources, avoiding processed egg products

Disclaimer: The elimination protocol can vastly differ according to the disease being treated. For instance, while treating a psychiatric disorder, we may not eliminate eggs or cheese which we would otherwise eliminate in the case of treating an autoimmune disorder. Similar is the case with nuts and seeds. Almonds, walnuts and peanuts might be eliminated while treating an autoimmune, cardiometabolic or digestive disorder. However, in case of treating a mental issue, these are permitted. All nuts and seeds, including almonds and walnuts, prevent or reduce neuroinflammation and are beneficial for neural and mental health and, therefore, are generally not excluded while following the elimination protocol. Hence, please consult a professional or your nutritionist before embarking on the elimination protocol.

Adding Beneficial Foods to Your Diet

Though we allow or disallow certain foods according to the disease and the patient's history, there are some common foods and ingredients which we usually add to the diet while we eliminate the potentially inflammatory foods. These are as follows:

➤ Herbs and Spices

Incorporating a variety of herbs and spices can enhance flavour and provide numerous health benefits. Here are some essential herbs and spices to include:

- **Celery leaves:** Rich in antioxidants and beneficial for reducing inflammation
- **Cilantro:** Known for its detoxifying properties, it helps to remove heavy metals from the body
- **Mint:** Aids in digestion and soothes the stomach
- **Ginger:** Contains powerful anti-inflammatory and antioxidant properties
- **Garlic:** Boosts the immune system and has antibacterial properties
- **Raw turmeric:** Contains curcumin, a potent anti-inflammatory compound
- **Basil:** Supports the immune system and has anti-inflammatory effects
- **Cumin:** Aids in digestion and is rich in iron
- **Cinnamon:** Helps regulate blood sugar levels and has anti-inflammatory properties

- **Lemongrass:** Known for its antioxidant and anti-inflammatory benefits
- **Nutmeg:** Supports digestion and has anti-inflammatory effects
- **Thyme:** Has antibacterial and antifungal properties
- **Rosemary:** Enhances memory and concentration, and has anti-inflammatory properties
- **Bay leaf:** Aids in digestion, and has antimicrobial properties
- **Oregano:** Contains antioxidants, and has antimicrobial effects
- **Asafoetida:** Helps with digestive issues, and has anti-inflammatory properties
- **Anise:** Supports digestion, and has antioxidant properties
- **Clove:** Contains eugenol, which has anti-inflammatory and pain-relieving properties
- **Mace:** Supports digestion, and has anti-inflammatory effects
- **Cardamom:** Aids in digestion, and has antioxidant properties
- **Fenugreek:** Helps regulate blood sugar levels, and has anti-inflammatory effects

➢ Fermented Foods

Fermented foods, as highlighted in the previous chapter, are rich in probiotics which promote a healthy gut microbiome. Including fermented foods in your diet can improve digestion, enhance nutrient absorption and boost the immune system. Some beneficial fermented foods include:

- **Kanji:** A traditional Indian fermented drink made from black carrots, beets and mustard seeds

- **Homemade Pickles:** Made with cold-pressed mustard oil and rock salt, free from artificial preservatives
- **Yogurt:** A rich source of probiotics, best when made from plant-based milks for those avoiding dairy
- **Kefir:** A fermented milk drink that is high in probiotics
- **Kimchi:** A Korean fermented vegetable dish that is rich in probiotics and vitamins
- **Sauerkraut:** Fermented cabbage that provides beneficial probiotics and fibre
- **Kombucha:** A fermented tea that contains probiotics and antioxidants

> **Nuts and Seeds**

Nuts and seeds are nutritional powerhouses that can play a significant role in enhancing mental well-being. Their rich reserves of essential fatty acids, vitamins, minerals and antioxidants support brain health, and can help alleviate symptoms of depression, anxiety and other mental health disorders.

- **Almonds:** High in vitamin E, magnesium and healthy fats. The magnesium in almonds helps manage stress and anxiety by regulating neurotransmitters and relaxing muscles. Vitamin E acts as an antioxidant, protecting the brain from oxidative stress.
- **Walnuts:** Rich in omega-3 fatty acids, antioxidants and polyphenols. Omega-3 fatty acids are crucial for brain function and development, and they have been shown to reduce symptoms of depression and improve cognitive function. The antioxidants in walnuts also help protect the brain from oxidative damage.
- **Cashews:** Contain magnesium, iron, zinc and healthy fats. The magnesium in cashews can help regulate

neurotransmitters involved in mood and relaxation. Zinc is essential for brain function and neuroplasticity, while iron is critical for oxygen transport to the brain.
- **Sunflower Seeds:** High in vitamin E, magnesium and selenium. Selenium is known for its mood-enhancing properties and ability to reduce inflammation. On the other hand, vitamin E supports brain health by protecting cells from oxidative stress.
- **Pumpkin Seeds:** Rich in magnesium, zinc, tryptophan and healthy fats. Tryptophan is a precursor to serotonin—a neurotransmitter that regulates the mood. Zinc supports cognitive function, and magnesium aids in stress reduction and relaxation.
- **Chia Seeds:** High in omega-3 fatty acids, fibre and antioxidants. Omega-3 fatty acids in chia seeds are vital for brain health and can help reduce symptoms of depression and anxiety. The high fibre content supports gut health, which is closely linked to mental health through the gut-brain axis.

Additional Nuts and Seeds

- **Flaxseeds:** High in omega-3 fatty acids and fibre; beneficial for brain health and gut health
- **Brazil Nuts:** Excellent source of selenium, which can improve mood and reduce inflammation
- **Hazelnuts:** Rich in vitamin E, which supports brain health and reduces oxidative stress

My firsthand experience with patients has shown that improving digestive and gut health and reducing neuroinflammation via the elimination protocol, along with the inclusion of herbs, spices and fermented foods in their diets, are significantly helpful in

*improving mood, cognition, mental acuity
and overall mental health.*

Additional Instructions for the Elimination Protocol

Sun Exposure

- Aim for at least 30 minutes of overhead sun exposure on bare skin, four times a week. This helps the body produce vitamin D, which is crucial for immune function and bone health.

Incorporating Healthy Fats

- Ensure you consume enough good fats in the form of ghee, mustard oil, nuts, seeds and butter. Healthy fats are essential for hormone production, brain health and overall cellular function.

Using Natural Salts

- Replace white table salt with coarse pink, black, sea or rock salt. These natural salts contain trace minerals that are beneficial for health.

Cooking Utensils

- Avoid using teflon or aluminium cookware which can release harmful chemicals. Instead use steel, clay pots, iron, copper or stone cookware—which are safer and can enhance the flavour of food.

Replacing Plastics

- Replace all plastics in the kitchen—including food containers and straws—with glass or steel alternatives.

Plastics can leach harmful chemicals into food, especially when heated.
- Avoid using styrofoam, silver foil and cling film. These materials can also release harmful substances into food, particularly when used with hot or acidic foods.

A Typical Timeline for the Elimination Phase

The elimination protocol typically spans three to four months, divided into two main phases:

1. **The First Six to Eight Weeks (Empiric Elimination of Common Food Allergens)**

    - The goal is to suppress active inflammatory markers. By removing potential allergens and inflammatory foods, the body can begin to heal and symptoms often start to improve.

2. **The Next Six to Eight Weeks (Maintaining Elimination and Monitoring Symptoms)**

    - This phase focuses on erasing immune memory cells such as NK cells to prevent the immune system from triggering inflammation upon the reintroduction of certain foods. This extended period ensures a more thorough reset of the body's immune response.
    - During this period, it's crucial to monitor symptoms closely to assess whether there is any improvement. This step is fundamental to providing the body with enough time to reduce inflammation and heal from any adverse reactions caused by these foods.
    - Patients are encouraged to:
        i. **Keep a Food Diary:** Record everything you eat and note any symptoms you experience.

ii. **Be Consistent:** Strictly avoid all eliminated foods to ensure accurate results.
iii. **Observe Changes:** Look for improvements in symptoms including reduced digestive discomfort, improved mental acuity, stable mood, calmer behaviour, clearer skin, improved respiratory function and decreased inflammation.

Phase II (The Reintroduction Phase)

After the elimination phase, foods are gradually reintroduced one at a time, every three to five days. This also requires the careful monitoring of any adverse reactions. Keeping a detailed journal of symptoms and reactions is crucial during this phase.

The Reintroduction Process

1. **Choose One Food Group:** Start with a single food group such as dairy.
2. **Reintroduce Gradually:** Consume a small amount of the food on the first day, and gradually increase the quantity over a few days.
3. **Monitor Symptoms and Assess Reactions:** During the reintroduction phase, we pay close attention to how your body responds to each food; keep a detailed record of any symptoms that arise during the reintroduction period. Symptoms to watch for include:
- Mental health behaviour (decreased focus, increased fidgetiness, the return of symptoms of anxiety and mood swings, lack of motivation, and so on)
- Digestive issues (bloating, gas, diarrhoea, constipation)
- Skin reactions (rashes, hives, eczema)
- Respiratory symptoms (congestion, asthma)

- General inflammation (joint pain, headaches, fatigue)

  If symptoms reappear during the reintroduction of a particular food, it is likely that this food is a trigger for the individual's symptoms. The particular food is then eliminated from the diet permanently to avoid adverse reactions. After the removal of a particular food, we wait until symptoms subside before reintroducing the next food.

4. **Wait and Observe:** We allow a few days after each reintroduced food group to ensure that any reactions are clearly linked to a specific food.

Simple Meal Plans

Embarking on the elimination protocol can seem daunting, but with careful planning and delicious recipes, it becomes manageable and even enjoyable. Here is a comprehensive meal plan that offers multiple options for each meal, ensuring variety and satisfaction while adhering to the principles of the elimination protocol.

Breakfast

- **Millet Porridge:** Made with ragi or jowar, topped with fresh fruit and a drizzle of honey
- **Smoothie:** Blended with spinach, banana, plant-based milk and a scoop of protein powder

Lunch

- **Quinoa Salad:** Mixed with vegetables, chickpeas and a lemon-tahini dressing
- **Grilled Chicken:** Served with a side of roasted vegetables and a millet-based grain like buckwheat

Dinner

- **Stir-fry:** Made with amaranth, fresh vegetables, tofu or tempeh, and a coconut aminos sauce
- **Bajra Roti:** Served with a hearty lentil soup and a side salad

Snacks

- **Fruit:** Fresh fruit such as green apples, berries or citrus
- **Nuts and Seeds:** Pumpkin seeds, sunflower seeds and chia seeds
- **Vegetable Sticks:** With homemade hummus or guacamole

Recipes

Let's look at a few recipes you can prepare at home with the ingredients allowed in the elimination protocol.

Breakfast Options

Option 1: Millet Porridge

Ingredients

- 1 cup ragi or jowar (millet) flour
- 2 cups water or coconut milk
- 1 tablespoon chia seeds
- Fresh berries or sliced banana
- A drizzle of honey or maple syrup (optional)

Recipe Instructions

- Mix millet flour with water or coconut milk in a pot.
- Cook over medium heat, stirring constantly, until it thickens.

- Stir in chia seeds and let it simmer for another 2-3 minutes.
- Serve with fresh berries or banana slices and a drizzle of honey or maple syrup.

Option 2: Smoothie Bowl

Ingredients

- 1 cup spinach
- 1 frozen banana
- ½ cup mixed berries
- 1 cup almond milk
- 1 tablespoon flaxseeds
- 1 tablespoon almond butter

Recipe Instructions

- Blend spinach, frozen banana, berries, almond milk, flaxseeds and almond butter until smooth.
- Pour into a bowl and top with fresh fruit, coconut flakes and additional seeds if desired.

Option 3: Quinoa Breakfast Bowl

Ingredients

- ½ cup cooked quinoa
- ¼ cup unsweetened coconut milk
- 1 tablespoon pumpkin seeds
- 1 tablespoon sunflower seeds
- Fresh fruit like green apple slices or blueberries

Recipe Instructions

- Warm the cooked quinoa in a pot with coconut milk.
- Transfer to a bowl and top with pumpkin seeds, sunflower seeds and fresh fruit.

Lunch Options

Option 1: Grilled Chicken Salad

Ingredients

- 1 grilled chicken breast, sliced
- Mixed greens (spinach, arugula, kale)
- ½ avocado, sliced
- Cherry tomatoes
- Cucumber slices
- Olive oil and lemon juice dressing

Recipe Instructions

- Combine mixed greens, avocado, tomatoes and cucumber in a bowl.
- Top with sliced grilled chicken.
- Drizzle with olive oil and lemon juice dressing.

Option 2: Lentil and Vegetable Soup

Ingredients

- 1 cup red lentils
- 1 carrot, diced
- 1 celery stalk, diced
- 1 onion, diced
- 2 cloves garlic, minced

- 4 cups vegetable broth
- 1 teaspoon turmeric
- 1 teaspoon cumin
- Fresh cilantro for garnish

Recipe Instructions

- In a large pot, sauté onion, garlic, carrot and celery until softened.
- Add lentils, vegetable broth, turmeric and cumin.
- Bring to a boil, then simmer for 20–25 minutes until lentils are tender.
- Garnish with fresh cilantro before serving.

Option 3: Quinoa and Vegetable Stir-Fry

Ingredients

- 1 cup cooked quinoa
- 1 bell pepper, sliced
- 1 zucchini, sliced
- 1 cup broccoli florets
- 2 tablespoons coconut aminos
- 1 tablespoon sesame oil
- 1 clove garlic, minced
- Fresh basil leaves

Recipe Instructions

- In a large pan, heat sesame oil and sauté the garlic until fragrant.
- Add bell pepper, zucchini and broccoli, and stir-fry until tender.

- Stir in cooked quinoa and coconut aminos.
- Garnish with fresh basil leaves before serving.

Mid-Day Snacking Options

Option 1: Fresh Fruit and Nut Butter

Ingredients

- Sliced green apple or pear
- 2 tablespoons almond or sunflower seed butter

Recipe Instructions

- Slice the apple or pear.
- Serve with a side of almond or sunflower seed butter for dipping.

Option 2: Hummus and Vegetable Sticks

Ingredients

- 1 cup homemade hummus (made from chickpeas, tahini, lemon juice, garlic and olive oil)
- Carrot sticks
- Celery sticks
- Cucumber slices

Recipe Instructions

- Prepare homemade hummus and place in a serving bowl.
- Serve with a variety of vegetable sticks for dipping.

Option 3: Chia Seed Pudding

Ingredients

- ¼ cup chia seeds
- 1 cup coconut milk
- 1 teaspoon vanilla extract
- Fresh berries or nuts for topping

Recipe Instructions

- Mix chia seeds, coconut milk and vanilla extract in a bowl.
- Refrigerate for at least two hours or overnight until it thickens.
- Top with fresh berries or nuts before serving.

Dinner Options

Option 1: Baked Salmon with Asparagus

Ingredients

- 1 salmon fillet
- 1 bunch asparagus
- 2 tablespoons olive oil
- 1 lemon, sliced
- Fresh dill
- Sea salt and black pepper to taste

Recipe Instructions

- Preheat oven to 375°F (190°C).
- Place salmon fillet and asparagus on a baking sheet.
- Drizzle with olive oil, season with sea salt and pepper, and top with lemon slices.

- Bake for 15–20 minutes until salmon is cooked through.
- Garnish with fresh dill before serving.

Option 2: Stuffed Bell Peppers

Ingredients

- 4 bell peppers, tops cut off and seeds removed
- 1 cup cooked quinoa
- 1 cup black beans, drained and rinsed
- 1 cup corn kernels
- 1 onion, diced
- 2 cloves garlic, minced
- 1 teaspoon cumin
- 1 teaspoon paprika

Recipe Instructions

- Preheat oven to 375°F (190°C).
- In a pan, sauté onion and garlic until softened.
- Add cooked quinoa, black beans, corn, cumin and paprika, and mix well.
- Stuff the bell peppers with the quinoa mixture and place them in a baking dish.
- Cover with foil and bake for 30–35 minutes.

Option 3: Zucchini Noodles with Pesto

Ingredients

- 2 large zucchinis, spiralized into noodles
- 1 cup fresh basil leaves
- ¼ cup pine nuts
- 2 cloves garlic

- ¼ cup olive oil
- 1 tablespoon nutritional yeast (optional)
- Sea salt and black pepper to taste

Recipe Instructions

- In a food processor, blend basil, pine nuts, garlic, olive oil, nutritional yeast, sea salt and black pepper until smooth.
- In a pan, lightly sauté the zucchini noodles until tender.
- Toss the zucchini noodles with the pesto sauce.
- Serve immediately.

Important Note

- Train yourself to listen to your body while being on the elimination protocol.
  - Pay close attention to how your body responds during the elimination and reintroduction phases.
  - Adjust the diet as needed based on the reactions observed.
- Consult a professional.
  - As already mentioned, you need to work with a nutritionist or healthcare provider to ensure that the elimination protocol is tailored to your specific needs and health conditions.

Nutritional and Lifestyle Interventions for a 42-Year-Old Woman

Five months ago, I met with a 42-year-old woman who was struggling with multiple health issues that significantly impacted her quality of life. When she first came to see me, she presented with a range of symptoms that had become increasingly unmanageable. She described her menstrual periods as irregular, sometimes occurring every 15 days for the past six to eight months. In addition to menstrual irregularities, she experienced muscle pain, spasms, unexplained fatigue and severe digestive issues, including bloating, pain, loss of appetite, diarrhoea and constipation.

Her mental health was also a concern; she was on Prozac but found it offered limited relief. She reported frequent allergies and intolerances, often experiencing wheezing and skin rashes. To manage her heavy menstrual bleeding, she was on Trapic MF. A blood test revealed that her cortisol levels were very high, indicative of extreme stress.

Her personal life was equally challenging. She had two young children, one of whom had special needs. She had no social support or time for herself as her husband, though a good man, was preoccupied with his business and unable to assist with childcare. The cumulative stress of managing her household and childcare responsibilities left her feeling overwhelmed and emotionally fragile.

Initial Assessment and Interventions

Upon reviewing her medical history, lifestyle and dietary habits, I decided to implement a comprehensive intervention plan. The first step was to address her dietary needs through an elimination diet protocol, which we followed for three months. This involved removing potential allergens and irritants from her diet to identify any food intolerances and reduce systemic inflammation.

While being on the elimination protocol, she was encouraged to eat home-made fermented foods and drinks. She alternately ate kimchi and drank kefir every day. I directed her to eat nutritionally dense food which included chia seed pudding and a homemade grilled chicken salad prepared from scratch (see recipes above).

Her dairy milk was substituted with almond and coconut milk. Additionally, she was asked to cook vegetables herself. I encouraged her to eat lentils, carrots, cruciferous vegetables and celery.

In addition to dietary changes, I prescribed a range of supplements to address her nutritional deficiencies and support her overall health. These included:

- **B Complex Vitamins**: To support energy production and reduce stress
- **Zinc**: To boost her immune system, improve skin health, and enhance cognition by strengthening neuroplasticity
- **Magnesium**: To alleviate muscle pain and spasms
- **Selenium**: For its antioxidant properties and thyroid function support
- **Folic Acid**: To support cell function and growth
- **Vitamin D**: To enhance mood and immune function
- **Tocopherol (Vitamin E) and Omega-3 Fatty Acids**: For their anti-inflammatory and antioxidant benefits, reducing neuroinflammation
- **L-Glutamine**: To support gut health and repair the intestinal lining
- **Probiotics**: To restore healthy gut flora and improve digestive health

Recognizing that her high stress levels were a significant factor in her health issues, I referred her to a professional counsellor for psychological support. I worked closely with her counsellor to suggest lifestyle interventions that would help her manage stress more effectively. These interventions included:

- Encouraging regular physical activity tailored to her energy levels

- Introducing relaxation techniques such as deep breathing exercises, meditation and yoga
- Establishing a more structured daily routine to create a sense of stability
- Promoting better sleep hygiene practices to improve the quality of her rest
- Encouraging her to carve out small pockets of time for self-care and hobbies she enjoyed

Progress and Outcomes

Over the course of the next five months, we monitored her progress closely. Her adherence to the elimination diet and supplement regimen was excellent, and she attended regular counselling sessions. The combined effect of these interventions led to significant improvements in her health.

Her menstrual cycles became regular, with her recent bloodwork showing normalized levels of progesterone, oestrogen, FSH (follicle-stimulating hormone), LH (luteinizing hormone), prolactin and insulin. She no longer required Prozac or antibiotics as her mental and physical health stabilized.

One of the most noticeable improvements was in her digestive health. She regained her appetite and no longer experienced severe bloating, pain, or the alternating phases of diarrhoea and constipation that previously plagued her. Her energy levels improved, and she reported feeling less fatigued and more capable of managing her daily responsibilities.

Emotionally, she became more resilient. The counselling sessions, combined with lifestyle changes, helped her develop better coping mechanisms for stress. She reported feeling more in control of her emotions and less likely to cry at the slightest provocation.

Conclusion and Reflection

By simultaneously addressing dietary needs, nutritional deficiencies and stress management, we were able to achieve significant improvements in her health and quality of life. This patient's journey highlights the importance of considering the interplay between physical, emotional and psychological factors in the management of chronic health issues.

Her case also serves as a reminder of the critical need for support systems for individuals caring for children with special needs. The stress and demands of such caregiving responsibilities can take a severe toll on a caregiver's health. Ensuring that they have access to appropriate resources and support is essential for their well-being.

The comprehensive and multidisciplinary approach we employed was key to her recovery. This experience reinforces my belief in the power of integrated care and the importance of addressing all aspects of a patient's life when devising a treatment plan. It was immensely gratifying to witness her transformation and know that the interventions we implemented had a lasting positive impact on her health and overall quality of life.

The Holistic Recovery of a 52-Year-Old Woman from Depression and Panic Attacks

Five months ago, a 52-year-old woman came to me seeking help for severe depression, anxiety and panic attacks. Her story was deeply touching and complex—involving a series of traumatic events that had taken a profound toll on her mental and physical health.

She lost her husband a few years ago, leaving her feeling alone and isolated. This emotional burden was compounded when she discovered a lump in her throat. Although her biopsy results came back normal, she became convinced she had throat cancer. This unfounded fear led to increased anxiety and ultimately caused her to stop dancing—an activity she once loved. As her anxiety grew, she developed gastric reflux; she either ate too much or too little. To cope with her emotional distress, she turned to alcohol which further exacerbated her gastric issues. She began to sweat excessively in her hands, and her anxiety intensified to the point where she experienced a panic attack, fainted and was hospitalized.

At the hospital, she was prescribed anti-depressants. However, despite these interventions, the lump in her throat persisted and neither antibiotics nor painkillers provided relief. It was clear that a more comprehensive approach was needed to address her health issues.

Initial Consultation and Interventions

Upon initial consultation, I recognized the need for a multidisciplinary approach. First, I connected her with a psychologist to begin cognitive-behavioural therapy (CBT). This therapy aimed to address her anxiety, depression and delusional thinking about the lump in her throat. Simultaneously, I designed a nutritional intervention plan to support her overall well-being.

Nutritional Interventions

1. **Vitamin and Mineral Supplementation**: I prescribed a regimen of essential vitamins and minerals to support her mental and physical health, including:
    - **Vitamin B6:** To help manage mood swings and improve brain function
    - **Folic Acid:** To support cognitive health and alleviate depressive symptoms
    - **Zinc:** For its role in neurotransmitter function and immune support

- **Magnesium:** To reduce anxiety and muscle tension
- **Selenium:** For its antioxidant properties and thyroid function support

2. **Herbal Supplements:** I included natural supplements known for their calming effects:
   - **Ashwagandha:** To reduce stress and anxiety
   - **5-HTP (5-Hydroxytryptophan):** As a precursor to serotonin, to improve mood and reduce anxiety; to be taken in the evening

3. **Dietary Elimination Protocol:** She followed this protocol to identify and eliminate potential neuroinflammatory foods and irritants from her diet, focusing on:
   - **Nutritionally Dense Foods:** Including nuts and seeds, Japanese seaweeds like nori and wakame, asparagus, and various Chinese leafy vegetables like Chinese cabbage, bok choy, napa cabbage and red cabbage
   - **Soy Methi:** Introduced for its potential health benefits
   - **Nut Milk:** Substituting dairy milk with almond milk and coconut milk to reduce inflammation and digestive discomfort
   - **Eliminating Alcohol and Caffeine:** To reduce anxiety and gastric reflux
   - **Substituting Refined Oils and Gluten-Based Foods:** With healthier options like coconut oil, desi ghee and millets

Progress and Recovery Phase

Over the next five months, we carefully monitored her progress. The combination of psychological counselling, dietary changes and nutritional supplementation brought about significant improvements in her mental and physical health.

1. Mental Health

The cognitive-behavioural therapy sessions helped her confront and manage her fears about the lump in her throat. Over time, she overcame her delusional thinking and stopped believing she had cancer. Her anxiety levels decreased, and she became more confident. She also stopped experiencing panic attacks, and with her doctor's guidance, was gradually weaned off her anti-depressants.

2. Digestive Health

The elimination diet and eating nutritionally dense foods significantly improved her digestive health. Her gastric reflux symptoms diminished, and she no longer experienced the discomfort that previously plagued her. Her eating habits stabilized and she maintained a balanced diet, avoiding the extremes of overeating and undereating.

3. Physical Health

The vitamins, minerals and herbal supplements supported her overall well-being. She reported feeling more energetic and less fatigued. The sweating in her hands subsided and her overall physical health improved.

4. Lifestyle Changes

After eliminating alcohol and caffeine from her diet, she noticed a marked improvement in her anxiety levels and digestive health. The substitution of refined oils and gluten-based foods with healthier options like coconut oil, desi ghee and millets contributed to the overall improvement of her health.

Conclusion and Reflection

By addressing the root causes of her anxiety and depression through psychological counselling and targeted nutritional interventions, we were able to bring about significant improvements in her mental and physical health. Her journey underscores the importance of considering all aspects of a patient's life when devising a treatment plan. The integration of cognitive-behavioural therapy with a tailored nutritional plan allowed her to regain control over her life, improve her mental clarity, and enhance her overall well-being.

Witnessing her transformation was incredibly rewarding. It highlighted the power of combining traditional medical approaches with holistic interventions to address complex health issues. This case reinforced my belief in the importance of a comprehensive approach to health, and the potential for recovery even in the face of significant challenges.

As she continues on her path to recovery, I remain committed to supporting her with ongoing nutritional guidance and lifestyle recommendations. Her resilience and progress serve as an inspiration, and I am confident that she will continue to thrive in her journey towards optimal health and well-being.

Managing ADHD through Nutrition and Therapy

A year ago, I began working with a 14-year-old boy from the United States—a non-resident Indian (NRI) patient who was brought to me with severe ADHD (attention-deficit hyperactivity disorder). His condition was particularly challenging due to his hyperactivity, inability to sit still, and constant fidgeting. Despite his parents' efforts—including the use of fidget-spinning toys—his hyperactivity remained uncontrolled. What caught my attention the most, however, were his persistent gut issues, alternating between constipation and diarrhoea, and his extremely dry skin which he would rub to the point of bleeding.

At the time of our initial consultation, he was on two ADHD medications and some homeopathic treatments. His parents had already eliminated milk and other dairy products from his diet in an attempt to address his gut issues, but this did not yield significant results. It was clear that a more comprehensive, integrated approach was needed to manage his ADHD symptoms and improve his overall well-being.

Initial Assessment and Collaborative Approach

Recognizing the complexity of his case, I decided to take a multidisciplinary approach. I partnered with a paediatric psychotherapist to address his hyperactivity through cognitive behavioural therapy (CBT), while I focused on his dietary needs.

The first step was to put him on an extensive elimination protocol. This approach involved the systematic removal of potential allergens, irritants and foods that could exacerbate his symptoms. The goal was to identify specific dietary triggers and provide his body with the nutrients needed to support brain function and gut health.

Dietary Interventions

The elimination protocol was comprehensive and rigorous. We removed the following from his diet:

- **Sugar-Based Products**: All forms of added sugars which are known to worsen hyperactivity and cause energy spikes and crashes
- **Wheat Flour and Wheat-Based Products**: To eliminate gluten, which can contribute to inflammation and gut issues in sensitive individuals

- **Nightshade Vegetables**: Including tomatoes, capsicums, potatoes, eggplants, peppers, and goji berries—which can trigger inflammation and worsen ADHD symptoms
- **Processed Foods**: Processed chicken nuggets, ham and bacon which often contain preservatives, additives and poor-quality fats
- **Junk Food and Refined Oils**: All forms of junk food and refined oils were eliminated, and he was encouraged to consume foods cooked in coconut oil instead

Having removed these foods, I introduced healthier, nutrient-dense alternatives to support his brain function and overall health:

- **Millets and Lentils**: These gluten-free grains and legumes provided a good source of fibre and sustained energy without causing spikes in blood sugar.
- **Good Fats**: Healthy fats were introduced through seeds, nut milk, olive oil, avocado and fatty fish. These fats are crucial for brain health and help to stabilize mood and behaviour.
- **Green Leafy Vegetables**: A variety of green leafy vegetables were included to provide essential vitamins, minerals and antioxidants.
- **Foods Rich in Neurotransmitters**: I specifically added foods that either contained or supported the production of neurotransmitters like acetylcholine, norepinephrine and melatonin—critical for focus, mood regulation and sleep. These included eggs, French beans, soybeans, kidney beans, peas, radish, pistachios, almonds, pineapples, fatty fish like salmon and sardines, mushrooms, and freshly prepared home-cooked chicken.

Progress and Observations

Within three months of starting the dietary intervention and CBT, the changes in my patient were remarkable.

- **Improved Sleep Quality**
  One of the earliest improvements we noticed was in his sleep patterns. The elimination of sugar and processed foods, combined with the introduction of melatonin-rich foods, helped him achieve more restful and consistent sleep. This, in turn, had a positive impact on his behaviour during the day.
- **Better Skin Health**
  His extremely dry skin began to improve as his diet became more balanced and rich in healthy fats. The introduction of good-quality fats like olive oil, coconut oil and avocado provided the essential fatty acids needed for skin health. Over time, the excessive skin rubbing and bleeding subsided.
- **Behavioural Stability**
  The combination of cognitive behavioural therapy and the elimination of inflammatory foods led to noticeable improvements in his behavioural stability. He became more focused during tasks, and his hyperactivity diminished. The structure provided by his new diet—including regular meals rich in nutrients—also contributed to his mental and physical stability.
- **Improved Mental Acuity**
  As his body adjusted to the new dietary regimen, his mental acuity sharpened. The inclusion of eggs, fatty fish and home-cooked chicken—foods rich in nutrients

essential for brain function—played a key role in enhancing his cognitive performance.

The Gradual Reintroduction of Dairy and Wheat

After the first three months of strict adherence to the elimination protocol, we began the process of reintroducing some form of dairy and wheat into his diet. This was done slowly and carefully, monitoring for any signs of relapse in his symptoms.

- **Dairy**: We started with small amounts of dairy products like yogurt and cheese, which are generally easier to digest than milk. His gut tolerated these well, and there were no adverse effects on his behaviour or skin.
- **Wheat**: Similarly, we introduced whole wheat products like bread and pasta in small amounts. Again, his body handled these reintroductions without any negative reactions.

By gradually reintroducing these foods, we were able to confirm that his body could handle them in moderation, provided his overall diet remained balanced and nutrient-dense.

Conclusion and Reflection

This case highlights the profound impact that dietary interventions can have on managing ADHD, particularly when combined with appropriate psychological therapies. The comprehensive elimination protocol not only helped to identify and eliminate dietary triggers but also provided the nutrients necessary to support my patient's brain function and overall health.

The success of this intervention also underscores the importance of a multidisciplinary approach in managing complex conditions like ADHD. Working closely with a paediatric psychotherapist allowed us to address both the psychological and physiological aspects of my patient's condition, leading to significant improvements in the quality of his life.

Reflecting on this journey, I am reminded of the power of food as medicine. By carefully selecting and balancing the nutrients my patient needed, we were able to bring about meaningful changes in his behaviour, mental acuity and physical health. His progress was encouraging and inspiring, and you will be happy to know that he now continues to thrive without any professional support.

Keep in Mind

The elimination protocol is a powerful tool in the quest for optimal health. By systematically removing and reintroducing foods, you can uncover hidden food sensitivities, reduce inflammation and improve overall well-being. With careful planning and a focus on whole, unprocessed foods, the elimination protocol can transform your relationship with food and pave the way for a healthier, happier life.

Following the elimination protocol does not mean sacrificing flavour or satisfaction. There are many variations of meal plans that can provide a variety of delicious and nutritious options that align with the protocol's guidelines. By incorporating these meals into your daily routine, you can support your health journey and discover which foods work best for your body. Remember to monitor your symptoms and consult a healthcare provider to ensure the elimination protocol is tailored to your specific needs.

8

Mindful Eating: Transforming How You Eat

Imagine savouring a symphony where each note, pause and melody is intertwined with the other to create an experience that transcends mere listening, turning into a euphoria you want to feel again. A meticulously orchestrated symphony takes you to a place deep inside yourself, and awakens those senses that help you connect with what makes you feel blissful and satisfied, as if a long-lasting thirst has been quenched. Similarly, mindful eating transforms the mundane act of consuming food into a harmonious interplay of your senses, awareness and nourishment.

In the fast-paced world where we live, meals are often consumed on the go, mindlessly devoured while multitasking, or hurriedly eaten in front of screens. This disconnection from the act of eating can lead to overeating, poor digestion and a lack of satisfaction. Mindful eating is an ancient practice that invites us to rekindle our relationship with food, fostering a deeper connection to the present moment and our bodies.

'The pleasure of the table belongs to all ages, to all conditions, to all countries, and to all areas; it mingles with all other pleasures, and remains at last to console us for their departure.'

—Jean Anthelme Brillat-Savarin

Up until this point, we have been focusing on what to eat and what not to because research studies have revealed that what we eat affects our health. What we do not understand much is how the way we eat also influences our health and well-being. Mindful thinking and eating, and enjoying life, are interrelated with food and meals. Sharing meals while eating together and paying our gratitude for the meal are a few of the ways by which one can feel significantly better.

As a nutritionist, I often liken mindful eating to a form of epicurean meditation—where each bite is savoured with the same reverence as one might accord to a masterpiece. It's about immersing oneself fully in the moment (being mindful), embracing the textures, flavours and aromas, and nurturing not just the body but also the mind and the soul. This approach not only fosters a healthier relationship with food but also enhances digestion and overall well-being.

We now introduce the concept of mindful eating, and explore how one can practise eating mindfully by engaging one's senses, eliminating distractions, and slowing down to allow the body to recognize fullness. Once you recognize fullness and find a deeper connection with the taste and quality of food, you will avoid overeating and not want to eat junk food, deep-fried food, or any other food of sub-standard quality.

Apart from eating healthy food, you can take your mental health and overall well-being a few notches higher with mindful eating. Imagine having a band with the best percussionists and string players, along with drums, violins, cellos and guitars of the best quality; but they are not playing the music in sync. *What will you experience?* They may sound good individually. However, being out of alignment, they will not provide you with the blissful experience you expected from them. This is where mindful eating comes in—to create a symphony and offer you the maximum benefits that you expect from foods rich in micronutrients, healthy fats and neurotransmitters.

Practical Implementation of Mindful Eating

1. Creating a Conducive Environment

The first step towards mindful eating is creating an environment that encourages mindfulness. This means eliminating distractions such as television, smartphones and even stressful conversations. Just as a painter needs a tranquil space to create art, your eating environment should be serene and free from interruptions. Set your table with care, perhaps with a candle or some calming music in the background. This signals your brain that it's time to focus solely on the meal before you.

2. Engaging All Senses

Engage all your senses before taking even the first bite. Observe the colours, shapes and arrangements of the food on your plate. Inhale deeply, taking in the aromas which can enhance the anticipation and enjoyment of the meal. Touch the food, if appropriate, feeling its texture. This multisensory engagement heightens your awareness and prepares the digestive system by triggering saliva production and enzyme secretion. Then, when you start eating, notice the sensations as you chew and savour each bite. This level of engagement from your senses will completely enhance the pleasure of eating and help you tune into your body's signals.

3. Practising Gratitude

This is perhaps the most important facet of practising mindful eating. Before eating, take a moment to appreciate the food in front of you. Consider the journey it has taken from farm to plate, and the efforts of those who have prepared it, and pay gratitude in your mind to those who made this journey possible—from farmer and truck driver, the vendor and retailer, to your spouse who eventually cooked it. This practice of gratitude can enhance your overall satisfaction and promote a positive emotional connection with your food, reducing the likelihood of overeating.

4. Eating Slowly

One of the cornerstones of mindful eating is slowing down. Chew each mouthful thoroughly, savouring the flavours and textures. This not only aids digestion but also allows your brain the time to register fullness, preventing overeating. Aim to chew each mouthful at least 20–30 times. Put down your utensils between bites, allowing yourself to fully experience each mouthful before moving on to the next.

5. Listening to Your Body

Tune in to your body's hunger and satiety cues. Begin eating when you're moderately hungry rather than ravenous, which can lead to overeating. Throughout the meal, periodically check in with yourself to assess your hunger levels. Aim to stop eating when you're comfortably satisfied, not stuffed. This practice cultivates a deeper connection with your body's needs, and fosters a healthier relationship with food.

6. Mindful Choices

Mindful eating also involves making conscious food choices that align with your health goals and ethical values. Choose foods that nourish your body and make you feel good. Pay attention to how different foods affect your energy levels and mood, and adjust your diet accordingly. This might mean opting for whole, unprocessed foods and being mindful of portion sizes.

7. Acknowledging Emotions

Food often becomes a coping mechanism for dealing with emotions. Mindful eating encourages recognizing and addressing these emotions without turning to food for comfort. Develop alternative strategies for managing stress, such as practising yoga, journalling, or talking to a friend. By addressing the root cause of emotional eating, you can build a healthier, more mindful approach to food.

8. Journalling about Your Experience

Keeping a mindful-eating journal can be an invaluable tool. Record what you eat, how you feel before and after meals, and any emotional triggers you notice. This practice can help you identify patterns and make more informed choices in the future. Over time, you'll become more attuned to your body's signals and develop a more intuitive approach to eating.

9. Mindful Snacking

Mindful eating isn't restricted to your main meals; it also applies to snacks. Approach snacking with the same level of mindfulness as full meals. Choose nutrient-dense snacks and savour them fully, rather than mindlessly munching on junk food. By doing so, you can maintain stable energy levels and avoid unnecessary weight gain.

10. Learning to Forgive Yourself

Mindful eating is not about perfection. There will be times when you eat mindlessly or overindulge. It's important to approach these moments with self-compassion rather than guilt. Recognize what happened, learn from it and move on. This forgiving attitude fosters a positive mindset and encourages long-term adherence to mindful eating practices.

11. Practising Mindful Cooking

The act of preparing food can also be a mindful practice. Engage fully in the process of cooking, from selecting ingredients to chopping vegetables and stirring the pot. Pay attention to the smells, sounds and colours as you cook. This not only enhances the pleasure of eating but also increases your appreciation for the food you prepare.

It is particularly useful when making probiotic-rich foods that involve fermentation. Fermentation is a time-honoured tradition that dates back thousands of years. By engaging in this practice, you connect with cultural and historical roots, preserving techniques passed down through generations. Fermenting at home allows you to appreciate the ancient wisdom and craftsmanship involved in creating these health-promoting foods.

Furthermore, the process of fermentation is a fascinating intersection of science and art. It involves understanding the roles of bacteria and yeast, maintaining optimal conditions for microbial growth, and observing the transformation of raw ingredients into complex, flavourful products. This hands-on experience fosters a deeper appreciation for the natural processes that sustain our health.

12. Community and Connection

Eating mindfully can also be a communal activity. Share meals with friends and family, savouring the experience together. Engage in meaningful conversations, but also take moments of silence to fully appreciate the food. This can strengthen relationships and create a more fulfilling dining experience.

When you become aware of how you're eating and find reverence for the food and its source, when you start honouring your hunger and satiety, and when you begin taking time to enjoy your food, you will discover that eating is a sacred experience with its own pleasure and privileges.

Mindful Hydration for Enhanced Cognitive Function

Staying hydrated is essential for maintaining optimal cognitive functions and overall well-being. However, many people underestimate the importance of drinking water mindfully and regularly—leading to issues like fatigue and stress. Dehydration can significantly impact your physical and mental health. When you don't drink enough water, your body struggles to perform essential functions, and this can manifest as:

- **Fatigue:** The lack of adequate hydration can lead to decreased energy levels, making you feel sluggish and tired. Your brain—which is about 75 per cent water—needs sufficient hydration to function effectively. Dehydration reduces its efficiency, leading to a decline in alertness and concentration.
- **Stress:** Dehydration increases the levels of the stress hormone cortisol in your body. This can exacerbate feelings of stress and anxiety, making it harder to cope with everyday challenges.

To combat these issues, it's important to drink water mindfully. Here's how you can do it:

1. **Set Hydration Goals:** Aim to drink at least eight glasses (about 2 litres) of water a day. Adjust this amount based on your activity level, the climate and individual needs.
2. **Carry a Water Bottle:** Keep a reusable water bottle with you throughout the day. This serves as a constant reminder to drink water and makes it convenient to sip frequently.
3. **Schedule Water Breaks:** Incorporate regular water breaks into your daily routine. Set reminders on your phone or use hydration apps to prompt you to drink water at regular intervals.
4. **Listen to Your Body:** Pay attention to signs of dehydration such as dry mouth, headaches or dark-coloured urine. These are signals that your body needs more water.
5. **Enhance Your Water:** If you find plain water boring, try infusing it with natural flavours like lemon, cucumber or mint. This can make drinking water more enjoyable and encourage you to drink more.

By staying hydrated, you can maintain better cognitive function, reduce fatigue, and manage stress more effectively. Remember, mindful hydration is a simple yet powerful tool to enhance your overall well-being and productivity. So make drinking water a priority and enjoy the benefits of a well-hydrated body and mind.

Basically, mindful eating is all about the meal process—from preparing the food and bringing it onto the table, to eating it and savouring it. Even the simplest foods can be pleasurable if we have a mindful attitude. We must enjoy the process of eating as it is as significant as the food we put in our body. Eating mindfully and with pleasure stimulates our whole body and overall health.

Rejuvenating a Life in Turmoil

When I first met 'Mr Anderson',[44] a 70-year-old widower, his physical and emotional state was deeply concerning. His journey to my care began under tragic circumstances—a fall that left him unconscious and unresponsive, leading to an urgent trip to the hospital. After being stabilized in the ICU, Mr Anderson was transferred to the general ward where the attending physician quickly noted signs of clinical depression. The root of this despair was painfully clear: the recent loss of his beloved wife—an event that left him emotionally shattered and physically debilitated.

Upon consultation with his family, I learnt that Mr Anderson was prescribed anti-depressants shortly after his wife's death. However, the medication did little to lift his spirits. He withdrew into himself, refusing to speak to hospital staff or engage with his family. He was malnourished, anorexic and frail—a shadow of the man he once was. His frailty likely contributed to his fall as he had become too weak from not eating or drinking adequately.

This was a man who lost not only his life partner but also his will to live. My role was clear: to help him regain his strength—both physical and emotional, and rediscover the joy that life still had to offer.

Initial Assessment and Nutritional Intervention

My first step was to address Mr Anderson's obvious malnutrition. His diet had become severely lacking in essential nutrients, which not only weakened his body but also exacerbated his depressive symptoms. I immediately directed his family to include nutritionally dense foods in his daily diet. These included:

---

[44] Name changed for privacy.

- **Dairy Products:** Curd and cheese—rich in calcium and probiotics—to strengthen his bones and improve his gut health
- **Healthy Fats:** Ghee and nuts like almonds and walnuts to provide him with essential fatty acids that support brain function and overall health
- **Vegetables and Lentils:** Green vegetables and lentils were included to ensure he received adequate fibre, vitamins and minerals
- **Legumes and Seeds:** Besan (chickpea flour) and various seeds like flaxseeds and chia seeds were introduced for their protein content and antioxidant properties

To address his micronutrient deficiencies, I prescribed a regimen of vitamin B complex supplements, along with other key micronutrients such as zinc and selenium. These are known to play a vital role in mental well-being, supporting cognitive function, and alleviating symptoms of depression.

The Inception of Gratitude and Mindful Eating

While the nutritional intervention was crucial, I knew that Mr Anderson's recovery also hinged on healing his wounded spirit. His grief was palpable, and his sense of loss left him disconnected from the world around him. To help him begin this emotional healing, I introduced the practice of gratitude as part of his daily routine—particularly at mealtimes.

Gratitude has profound effects on mental health, fostering a positive outlook and promoting emotional resilience. I encouraged Mr Anderson to focus on the blessings that still remained in his life, even amidst his profound loss. His family, especially his grandchildren who adored him, became the cornerstone of this practice. Each meal became an opportunity for Mr Anderson to reflect on the love and joy they brought into his life, and express gratitude for the nourishing food prepared with care by his family.

This practice of gratitude was intertwined with mindful eating—a simple yet powerful approach to food that involves engaging all the senses. I encouraged Mr Anderson to savour each bite, notice the textures, flavours and aromas of the food, and appreciate the effort that went into preparing it. His family played a vital role in this process, creating a warm and supportive environment at mealtimes. The dining table became a place not just for nourishment, but for connection, conversation and healing as well.

Results: A Remarkable Transformation

The transformation that followed was nothing short of remarkable. Within six weeks of starting the programme, Mr Anderson's physical health showed significant improvement. The weight he lost due to malnutrition was regained, and he began to develop lean muscle mass. His frailty was replaced by a newfound strength and vitality.

However, the most heartening change was in his mental and emotional states. As he continued the practice of gratitude and mindful eating, Mr Anderson slowly emerged from the fog of depression. The man who once withdrew into silence became more talkative, engaging with his family and medical staff with a warmth and openness that was absent for months. He began to laugh and play with his grandchildren, finding joy in their presence and a renewed sense of purpose in his role as their grandfather.

The improvement in his mood and overall well-being was so significant that his doctor was able to take him off the antidepressants. Mr Anderson found a way to heal that went beyond medication—he reconnected with the simple pleasures of life, the love of his family, and the joy of living in the present moment.

A New Chapter of Life

Reflecting on Mr Anderson's journey, I am struck by the resilience of the human spirit. What began as a desperate struggle for survival became a story of renewal and hope. Through the power of nutrition, the practice of gratitude and the simple act of mindful eating, Mr Anderson was able to reclaim his health and his happiness. He is now living each day with a newfound appreciation for life and the people who make it meaningful. His journey reminds us that healing is not just about treating symptoms, but also about nurturing the mind, body and soul.

Mr Anderson's story is a testament to the enduring power of love, connection, and the small, mindful choices we make each day. As he continues to enjoy his meals surrounded by family, each bite is a celebration of life—a life that, despite its losses, still holds the promise of joy, love and contentment.

Keep in Mind

Mindful eating is a transformative practice that extends beyond the plate. It fosters a deeper connection with our food, our bodies and our overall well-being. By creating an environment conducive to mindful eating, engaging our senses, practising gratitude, eating slowly, and listening to our bodies, we can cultivate a mindful eating practice that nourishes both body and soul. Embracing mindful choices, acknowledging emotions, journalling, and engaging in mindful snacking, self-forgiveness, mindful cooking and communal eating further enrich this practice. Ultimately, mindful eating is about making each meal an opportunity for nourishment, gratitude and joy, turning the act of eating into a celebration of life itself.

9

Intuitive Eating: Awakening the Body's Wisdom

Flashback—remember, we discussed the dopamine connection to processed food. When we eat foods high in sugar, trans fats and salt, common characteristics of processed foods, our brain's reward system is activated, stimulating dopamine release. This intense dopamine response—'dopamine rush'—leads to cravings and overeating as the brain seeks more pleasurable sensations associated with processed foods. However, what we did not discuss was how to prevent it. Well, in Part 2, we examined the answer to this question. But there is more to it when it comes to tackling a dopamine rush.

Intuitive eating is a revolutionary approach to nutrition and self-care that emphasizes trusting and listening to your body's internal cues, rather than external diet rules. Originating from the need to combat the adverse effects of diet culture and restrictive eating, intuitive eating promotes a healthy relationship between food, the mind and the body. Practising this daily becomes a measure to counter overeating processed food or overeating altogether. It helps individuals distinguish between experiencing a dopamine rush and actual satisfaction, enabling them to break free from the cycle of mindless overeating, and embrace a more balanced and fulfilling approach to nourishment. We will now delve into the history and origins of intuitive eating, outlining its core principles and providing practical guidelines for incorporating intuitive eating into daily life.

The History and Origin of Intuitive Eating

Intuitive eating was conceptualized in 1995 by dietitians Evelyn Tribole and Elyse Resch. They published the book *Intuitive Eating: A Revolutionary Program that Works* in response to rising concerns about the negative impacts of dieting. Tribole and Resch observed that dieting often led to a cycle of weight loss and gain, increased food obsession, and disordered eating patterns. Their approach sought to break this cycle by fostering a healthy relationship between food and the body.

The Problem with Diet Culture

Diet culture—which promotes thinness as the pinnacle of health and beauty—has been pervasive for decades. It often encourages restrictive eating, calorie counting, and food moralizing (labelling foods as 'good' or 'bad'). This culture can lead to harmful behaviours such as binge eating, emotional eating and chronic dieting, which negatively impact both physical and mental health.

The Birth of Intuitive Eating

Tribole and Resch's intuitive eating framework emerged as an antidote to diet culture. It focuses on internal bodily cues such as hunger and fullness, rather than external rules. This approach encourages individuals to trust their bodies, make peace with food, and prioritize self-care. Intuitive eating aligns with a holistic view of health—encompassing physical, mental and emotional well-being.

The 10 Principles of Intuitive Eating

Intuitive eating is built on 10 foundational principles designed to guide individuals towards a more mindful and self-compassionate approach to eating. Each principle addresses a specific aspect of eating behaviour and self-perception, promoting a balanced and healthy relationship with food.

1. Reject the Diet Mentality

The first principle urges individuals to reject the false promises of dieting. Diets often offer temporary solutions and unrealistic expectations that can lead to disappointment and a sense of failure. Rejecting the diet mentality means letting go of the belief that there is a 'perfect' diet or quick fix for weight loss. This principle encourages individuals to recognize and challenge messages from diet culture, whether they come from the media, social networks, or even healthcare professionals. By rejecting these messages, individuals can start to trust their own bodies and focus on long-term health rather than short-term weight loss.

2. Honour Your Hunger

This principle emphasizes the importance of recognizing and responding to the biological signals of hunger. Honouring your hunger means paying attention to your body's hunger cues and eating when you are truly hungry. Ignoring these signals can lead to intense cravings and overeating. By respecting your hunger, you can maintain your body's natural balance and prevent the cycle of restriction and bingeing.

3. Make Peace with Food

Making peace with food involves giving yourself the unconditional permission to eat, and removing the power struggle around food choices. This principle encourages individuals to eliminate food restrictions and stop labelling foods as 'good' or 'bad'. By allowing all foods in moderation, you reduce the guilt and anxiety associated with eating certain foods. This approach helps to normalize eating patterns and fosters a healthier relationship with food.

4. Challenge the Food Police

The food police are the critical voices that monitor your eating and judge your food choices. Challenging the food police means rejecting the internal and external critics enforcing diet rules. This principle encourages you to silence guilt-inducing thoughts and embrace a more compassionate attitude towards yourself. By doing so, you can focus on nourishing your body without judgement or self-criticism.

5. Discover the Satisfaction Factor

This principle highlights the importance of finding joy and satisfaction in eating. Eating should be a pleasurable experience—not just a means to an end. By choosing foods that you enjoy and eating in a pleasant environment, you can enhance your eating experience and feel more satisfied. This satisfaction can reduce the desire to overeat and improve your overall well-being.

6. Feel Your Fullness

Feeling your fullness involves paying attention to your body's signals that indicate that you are no longer hungry. This principle encourages mindful eating, where you listen to your body's cues for fullness, and stop eating when you feel comfortably satisfied. By doing so, you can avoid overeating and maintain a healthy balance. It requires slowing down, eating without distractions and checking in with your hunger levels throughout the meal.

7. Cope with Your Emotions with Kindness

Emotional eating is a common response to stress, boredom or other emotions. This principle addresses healthier ways to cope with emotions. Instead of turning to food for comfort, this principle encourages you to find alternative ways to manage your emotions, such as engaging in physical activity, practising mindfulness, or seeking support from others. Recognizing the emotional triggers for eating and addressing them directly can help break the cycle of emotional eating, and promote mental health.

8. Respect Your Body

Respecting your body means accepting your natural shape and size, and appreciating what your body does for you. This principle encourages body positivity and self-acceptance. By respecting your body, you can focus on health-promoting behaviours, rather than striving for an unrealistic body ideal. This shift in perspective helps to build self-esteem and encourages a more compassionate and holistic approach to self-care.

9. Movement—Feel the Difference

This principle promotes the idea of engaging in physical activity for pleasure and health, rather than as a means to lose weight. Movement should be enjoyable and something that makes you feel good. This principle encourages you to find physical activities that you enjoy and that make you feel energized. By focusing on how the movement feels rather than its calorie-burning potential, you can develop a more positive relationship with exercise and maintain an active lifestyle.

10. Honour Your Health with Gentle Nutrition

The final principle emphasizes making food choices that honour your health and taste buds while making you feel good. Gentle nutrition means choosing foods that are both nourishing and satisfying. It involves a balanced approach to eating that prioritizes whole, nutrient-dense foods while also allowing for the occasional treat. This principle encourages a flexible and sustainable approach to eating that supports overall health and well-being.

Practical Guidelines for Implementing Intuitive Eating

Transitioning to intuitive eating requires time, patience and practice. Here are some practical guidelines to help you incorporate the principles of intuitive eating into your daily life:

1. Self-Reflection and Awareness

Start by reflecting on your current eating habits and relationship with food. Journalling can be a helpful tool for this process. Write down your thoughts and feelings about food and body image. Identify any diet rules or beliefs you currently hold. Awareness is the first step towards change.

2. Mindful Eating Practices

Practise mindful eating by paying full attention to your eating experience. Eat without distractions such as TV or smartphones. Take the time to savour each bite, notice the flavours, and chew slowly. This practice helps you tune into your hunger and fullness cues.

3. Meal Planning with Flexibility

Plan meals that include a variety of foods you enjoy while being flexible and open to changes. Create balanced meals that include proteins, carbohydrates, fats and vegetables. Let yourself adjust your plan based on your hunger and cravings. Flexibility is key to maintaining a positive relationship with food.

4. Address Emotional Eating

Develop alternative coping strategies for managing emotions. Identify non-food activities that help you cope with stress, boredom or other emotions, such as walking, meditating or talking to a friend. Practise these activities regularly to build new habits.

5. Physical Activity for Enjoyment

Engage in physical activities that you find enjoyable and fulfilling. Explore different types of exercise such as dancing, hiking, swimming or yoga. Choose activities that make you feel good and look forward to doing them regularly.

6. Seek Support

Surround yourself with a supportive community, or seek professional help if needed. Join intuitive eating support groups—either in-person or online. Consider working with a registered dietitian or therapist who specializes in intuitive eating to guide you through the process.

7. Practise Self-Compassion

Be kind and patient with yourself as you transition to intuitive eating. Acknowledge that change takes time and that it's normal to encounter challenges along the way. Celebrate small victories and learn from setbacks without judgement.

8. Educate Yourself

Learn more about intuitive eating and the principles behind it. Read books, listen to podcasts and follow reputable sources on intuitive eating. Knowledge can empower you to make informed decisions and reinforce your commitment to this approach.

9. Focus on Long-Term Health

Prioritize long-term health and well-being over short-term weight loss. Shift your focus from achieving a certain weight or body size to improving overall health. Adopt habits that enhance your physical, mental and emotional well-being.

10. Celebrate Your Journey

Recognize and celebrate your progress in developing a healthier relationship with food. Reflect on the positive changes you've made and the benefits you've experienced. Celebrate your journey towards intuitive eating as a continuous and evolving process.

Keep in Mind

Intuitive eating offers a transformative approach to nutrition and self-care that rejects diet culture and promotes a healthy, balanced relationship between food and the body. By understanding its history, embracing its 10 principles, and following practical guidelines, you can cultivate a more mindful, compassionate and sustainable approach to eating. You must embrace intuitive eating to experience the joy it brings to your relationship with food.

A Note on the Subtle Differences between Mindful Eating and Intuitive Eating

Mindful eating and intuitive eating are two approaches that aim to cultivate a healthier relationship with food, but they differ in their focus and methodology. Understanding these differences can provide individuals with valuable insights into choosing the approach that aligns best with their needs and goals.

Mindful eating is rooted in the practice of mindfulness which involves being fully present and aware of one's thoughts, feelings and sensations in the moment without judgement. When applied to eating, mindfulness encourages individuals to pay attention to the entire eating experience: from selecting food and chewing slowly, to experiencing the flavours and textures, and recognizing satiety cues. The emphasis is on being mindful of the process of eating itself, promoting a deeper connection with food, and fostering a heightened awareness of hunger and fullness signals. Mindful eating often incorporates elements of meditation and self-reflection to enhance awareness and reduce mindless or emotional eating habits.

By contrast, intuitive eating is a broader philosophy that goes beyond the act of eating to encompass one's entire relationship with food and one's body. Developed by dietitians Evelyn Tribole and Elyse Resch, intuitive eating is based on 10 principles that encourage individuals to reject diet culture, honour hunger and fullness cues, and trust their body's wisdom to guide their eating choices. Unlike mindful eating, intuitive eating is not solely focused on the present moment, but also emphasizes the importance of rejecting external food rules, cultivating body acceptance, and addressing emotional and psychological factors that influence eating behaviours. It encourages individuals to rely on the internal cues of hunger, satiety and satisfaction, rather than external cues such as calorie counting or food restrictions.

One key difference between mindful eating and intuitive eating lies in their scope and underlying principles. Mindful eating is primarily concerned with the practice of mindfulness applied to eating, promoting awareness and presence during meals to enhance overall well-being. On the other hand, intuitive eating is a comprehensive approach that encompasses a broader set of principles aiming to rebuild a healthy relationship with food and body image over the long term. While both approaches advocate for tuning into bodily signals and reducing distractions during meals, intuitive eating also addresses the societal and psychological factors that influence eating behaviours and body perception.

Additionally, the practices associated with each approach may differ in their application. Mindful eating often involves specific techniques such as guided meditations, sensory awareness exercises, and paying deliberate attention to eating rituals. In contrast, intuitive eating encourages individuals to explore and understand their unique hunger and fullness cues without judgement or restriction, fostering a more flexible and sustainable approach to eating habits.

In summary, while both mindful eating and intuitive eating promote a healthier approach to food consumption, they differ in focus and methodology. Mindful eating emphasizes the practice of mindfulness during meals to enhance awareness and reduce mindless eating, whereas intuitive eating encompasses a broader philosophy that encourages rejecting diet culture, honouring internal cues, and nurturing a positive relationship between food and the body. Choosing between these approaches depends on individual preferences, goals and the desired depth of engagement with one's eating habits and overall well-being.

A Few Last Words

As we reach the end of this journey, I want to speak to you from the heart. The insights and strategies shared in this book are more than just information—they are pathways to a healthier, happier life. My hope is that you feel inspired and empowered to make positive changes in your diet that will enhance your mental well-being.

If you are struggling with mental health challenges or feel lost in the chaos of life, I hope the case studies in this book instill a sense of hope in you. Healing is possible. Through mindful dietary and lifestyle changes, you can regain clarity, balance and inner peace.

We live in a world where convenience often leads us towards highly processed foods, but the cost to our mental and physical health is too great. Regular consumption of refined sugars and unhealthy oils can take a significant toll on our mood and overall well-being. Instead, let us return to the nourishment that nature provides. Home-cooked meals prepared with care and intention offer a wealth of nutrients that our bodies and minds truly need.

Consider making small, mindful shifts in your eating habits. Move away from refined oils and sugars, and embrace healthier alternatives like coconut oil and olive oil which provide beneficial fats that support brain function. Incorporate nutrient-rich foods—leafy greens, nuts, seeds and fresh fruits—that help boost neurotransmitter production and elevate your mood.

I understand that changing long-standing habits is not easy, and I want you to know that you are not alone in this journey. Start with small, manageable steps. Practise mindful eating—savour each bite, appreciate the flavours, and recognize the nourishment it brings. Listen to your body, honour its needs, and treat it with kindness and respect.

Your mental health is precious, and the foods you choose to eat play a vital role in supporting it. I hope you find joy in preparing and enjoying wholesome, nutritious meals. May your path be filled with vibrant health, boundless energy, and a deep sense of well-being.

Thank you for allowing me to be part of your journey. Wishing you happiness, health and mindful eating—now and always.

Acknowledgements

This book marks another milestone in my professional journey as a nutritionist—a testament to years of research, learning and countless interactions with those seeking to heal through food. It reflects my deep belief in the power of nutrition, not only in shaping our physical health but also in influencing our mental well-being.

First and foremost, I wish to acknowledge my beloved late mother, whose nurturing spirit and unwavering faith in the power of nourishment ignited my passion for nutrition. From a young age, she instilled in me the value of wholesome, quality food as the foundation of good health. Her love and wisdom continue to guide me, shaping every step of my journey.

I am also deeply grateful to my father, whose stories—shared with such warmth and passion—have been a source of inspiration through the highs and lows of my career. His steadfast encouragement has been my anchor through life's challenges, reminding me of the importance of resilience and curiosity.

Lastly, to my incredible husband—my greatest champion and confidant—thank you for your unwavering patience, love and understanding. Through every late night, every draft and every challenge, your steadfast support has given me the strength to pursue this work. Your belief in my dreams has fuelled my determination to push boundaries in my field. This book, like all the others, is as much yours as it is mine.

Index

acetylcholine (ACh), 25, 120
Alzheimer's disease (AD), 25, 64, 65, 67, 135
analgesics, 45, 46
anxiety, xi, xiii, 5, 9, 11, 16, 18, 19, 20, 21, 23, 25, 29, 50, 52, 60, 62, 66, 71, 72, 74, 75, 89, 90, 91, 94, 95, 97, 102, 105, 116, 119, 120, 121, 132, 142, 149, 150, 157, 158, 161, 174, 175, 176, 177, 178, 190, 199
ashwagandha, 141
attention-deficit hyperactivity disorder (ADHD), 25, 26, 64, 65, 135, 178, 179, 180, 182
autism, 16, 21, 72, 73

binge, 64, 197, 198
brain-derived neurotrophic factor (BDNF), 66, 67, 80, 103, 122, 127, 134, 135

cardiovascular diseases (CVDs), 6, 39, 95

cerebral palsy, 65
cognitive-behavioural therapy (CBT), 175, 177, 178, 179, 181
cortisol, xiii, 8, 9, 15, 16, 71, 90, 171, 190
cortisol dysregulation, 9
C-reactive protein (CRP), 32, 50, 105

dietary fibres, 8, 88, 101
dopamine, xii, 7, 8, 11, 12, 13, 16, 19, 21, 22, 28, 40, 60, 66, 80, 89, 92, 118, 123, 124, 125, 126, 128, 130, 131, 134, 140, 142, 145, 196

elimination protocol, 148, 149, 150, 151, 154, 155, 158, 160, 162, 163, 170, 171, 179, 182, 183
endorphins, xii, 70, 74, 92, 124, 126, 134
enteric nervous system (ENS), 13, 14, 28, 53, 141

fermented foods, 96, 100, 101, 102, 103, 104, 107, 108, 143, 146, 149, 156, 158, 171
FODMAP, 57, 58, 59
folate (Vitamin B9), 91, 117, 122, 123, 145

gamma-aminobutyric acid (GABA), 7, 12, 13, 16, 19, 22, 23, 24, 28, 29, 52, 60, 66, 72, 80, 115, 120, 124, 125, 129, 130, 132, 133, 138, 141, 145
glutamate, 11, 66, 70, 73, 80, 124, 126, 128, 130, 132, 133, 137, 145
glutamic acid or glutamine, 128, 129, 130, 138
gut-associated lymphoid tissue (GALT), 100
gut-brain axis, xii, xiii, xiv, 7, 8, 10, 12, 13, 14, 15, 16, 17, 18, 27, 28, 50, 69, 76, 86, 90, 96, 115, 123, 130, 131, 149, 158
gut dysbiosis, 14, 32, 35, 41, 53, 55, 60, 66, 77, 80, 149, 150
gut microbiota, 7, 13, 14, 15, 16, 18, 19, 20, 28, 32, 41, 45, 46, 48, 50, 51, 52, 53, 55, 77, 83, 88, 96, 97, 99, 100, 102, 116, 129, 149

histamines, 70, 74, 75, 139
hypothalamic-pituitary-adrenal (HPA) axis, 89

inflammation, xiii, xiv, 8, 32, 33, 34, 39, 41, 46, 47, 50, 51, 53, 54, 57, 60, 64, 65, 66, 67, 68, 69, 76, 77, 82, 84, 89, 91, 94, 95, 100, 101, 104, 105, 115, 127, 133, 145, 147, 148, 149, 150, 152, 155, 158, 160, 161, 162, 171, 176, 179, 180, 183
intestinal fatty acid-binding protein (I-FABP), 67
intuitive eating, xii, xiv, 14, 196, 197, 198, 201, 202, 203, 204, 205
iron, 55, 92, 103, 121, 140, 145, 155, 157, 158, 159
irritable bowel syndrome (IBS), 23, 149

L-DOPA, 126, 130, 131, 140
leaky gut, xii, xiii, xiv, 7, 8, 32, 33, 34, 35, 36, 38, 46, 47, 48, 50, 51, 53, 61, 62, 65, 66, 68, 75, 76, 77, 80, 84, 87, 103,

105, 127, 130
Low-Carb/High-Fat Diet, 104

mindful eating, xiv, 80, 106, 184, 185, 186, 187, 188, 189, 191, 194, 195, 199, 201, 204, 205, 207

neuroinflammation, xiv, 66, 89, 122, 125, 135, 154, 158, 172
norepinephrine, 11, 19, 24, 25, 26, 28, 30, 122, 123, 128, 130, 131, 140, 180
NSAIDs (nonsteroidal anti-inflammatory drugs), 46

obsessive-compulsive disorder (OCD), 21, 65
omega-3, xiv, 38, 39, 72, 117, 118, 133, 134, 135, 141, 145, 157, 158
omega-6, 38, 39, 42, 95, 133
opioids, 36, 46, 47
oxytocin, xii, 70, 71, 72, 92, 124, 139

Parkinson's disease, 11, 64, 65, 119, 140
phenylalanine, 126, 131
post-traumatic stress disorder (PTSD), 21, 72
prebiotics, xiv, 81, 82, 83, 86, 87, 88, 90, 91, 94, 96, 114, 115, 146
prebiotics, 83, 86, 87, 90, 146
probiotics, xiv, 8, 42, 44, 45, 48, 51, 59, 77, 81, 82, 83, 84, 86, 87, 88, 90, 98, 99, 102, 104, 107, 108, 112, 115, 143, 145, 146, 149, 156, 157, 193
protein putrefaction, 41
proton pump inhibitor (PPI), 55

SAM (S-adenosylmethionine), 123, 131
schizophrenia, 5, 21, 73, 75, 121, 122
seasonal affective disorder (SAD), 26, 36, 37, 38, 42
selenium, 93, 121, 158, 193
serotonin, xii, 7, 8, 11, 12, 13, 15, 16, 19, 21, 28, 52, 60, 66, 76, 80, 82, 89, 92, 115, 117, 120, 121, 122, 123, 124, 125, 128, 131, 132, 134, 139, 140, 142, 145, 150, 158, 176
small intestinal bacterial overgrowth (SIBO), 55, 56, 57, 58, 60, 77, 83, 84, 140
symbiotic culture of bacteria and yeast (SCOBY), 99, 112

trans fats, 8, 37, 40, 41, 42, 48, 95, 196
triglycerides, 101, 152
tryptophan, 15, 20, 66, 122, 129, 158
type 2 diabetes, 101
tyrosine, 42, 122, 129, 131

vitamin B2, 124
vitamin B3, 125
vitamin B5, 125
vitamin B6, 92, 145
vitamin B12, 117, 131
vitamin C, 72, 93, 95
vitamin D3, 117, 118
vitamin E, 145, 157, 158

zinc, 103, 105, 117, 118, 121, 140, 141, 157, 158, 193